FIREFIGHTER'S FITNESS HANDBOOK

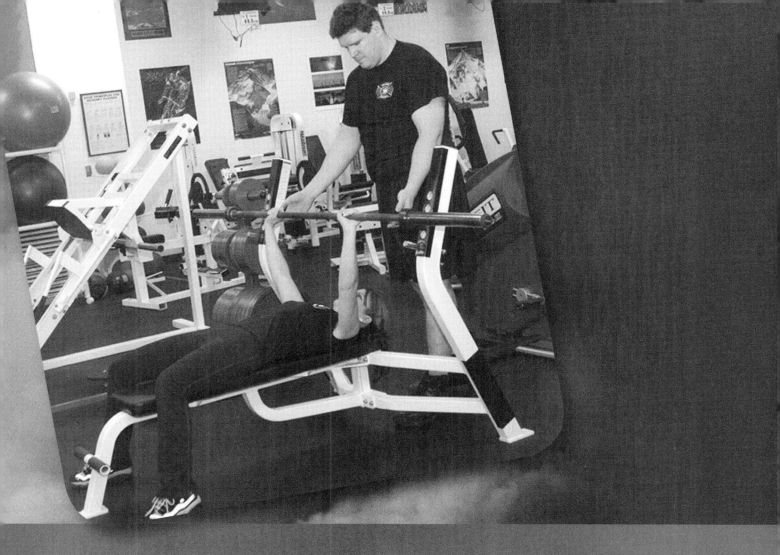

FIREFIGHTER'S FITNESS HANDBOOK

Al Wasser
Andrea Walter

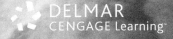
DELMAR
CENGAGE Learning

Australia • Brazil • Japan • Korea • Mexico • Singapore • Spain • United Kingdom • United States

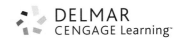

DELMAR
CENGAGE Learning™

Firefighter's Fitness Handbook
First Edition
Al Wasser
Andrea Walter

Vice President, Career and Professional Editorial: David Garza

Director of Learning Solutions: Sandy Clark

Product Development Manager: Janet Maker

Managing Editor: Larry Main

Editorial Assistant: Amy Wetsel

Production Director: Wendy Troeger

Production Manager: Mark Bernard

Marketing Director: Deborah Yarnell

Marketing Manager: Erin Coffin

Marketing Coordinator: Shanna Gibbs

Art Director: Benj Gleeksman

Compositor: PrePressPMG

Cover Designer: PrePressPMG

Cover Image: Stuart Dee/Getty Images

Library of Congress Control Number: 2008942165

ISBN-13: 978-1-4283-6148-5

ISBN-10: 1-428-36148-0

Delmar
5 Maxwell Drive
Clifton Park, NY 12065-2919
USA

Cengage Learning products are represented in Canada by Nelson Education, Ltd.

For your lifelong learning solutions, visit **delmar.cengage.com**.

Visit our corporate website at **www.cengage.com**

Notice to the Reader

Printed in Canada
1 2 3 4 5 6 7 8 9 12 09 08

Dedication

This book is dedicated to every firefighter that has laced up his or her athletic shoes, lifted weights, exercised, or made healthy nutritional choices because it impacts the way the job of firefighting gets done. When you make a commitment to improve your fitness and health, you do it for yourself, your safety, and the safety of your fellow firefighters.

Thank you for the work that you do every day, both to protect your community and to protect yourself.

Contents

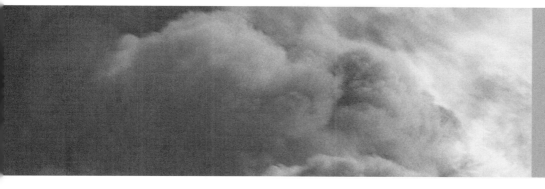

1

Health and Fitness of Firefighters   1

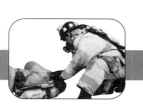

2

The Four Success Principles   12

3

Learning the Skills   22

4

Planning Your Workouts   62

5

Creating a Healthy Culture   86

Preface

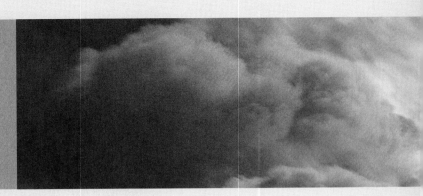

The *Firefighter Fitness Handbook* is for current and prospective firefighters and firefighter candidates who are interested in staying fit and healthy to perform their best as firefighters and, most importantly, to stay safe. This manual is also for the fire science instructor who wishes to include a firefighter fitness course in the curriculum. As a part of the fire science curriculum, the *Firefighter Fitness Handbook* can be used as a companion to the *Firefighter's Handbook Series* from Delmar Cengage Learning in order to help incoming candidates learning fundamental firefighting skills also expand their knowledge of health and fitness and how it impacts their skill performance.

Every year, firefighter fatality statistics consistently show that firefighters are dying from heart attacks at a much higher rate than are people in other occupations. Maintaining an individual's fitness and health is one of the most important activities that can be done to keep firefighters safe on the job, while improving their performance. The benefits to individual firefighters are overwhelming in scope, yet there is still a long way to go to ensure that every firefighter is establishing and working towards fitness and health goals.

To address this need, the fire science community developed the Joint Labor/Management Wellness-Fitness Initiative (WFI) in 1996. This manual utilizes the standards set forth in the initiative and also incorporates the principles from NFPA 1583 and the Life Safety Initiatives.

CONCEPTUAL APPROACH TO WRITING THIS BOOK

This book first came about as a result of initiatives to improve the coverage of physical fitness and health in the *Firefighter's Handbook*. The authors felt that as the statistics became more and more consistent in firefighter fatalities, the coverage of fitness and health deserved the attention of a full book and not just a few paragraphs. The next step was to partner with fitness experts that designed the *Mastering the CPAT* book, since the CPAT test is based on firefighter on-the-job skills. From there, the focus was on how to help firefighters in all types of departments set and meet goals for fitness and health improvement. The paramount goal from this is the improved safety and health of firefighters across the nation.

One of the underlying concepts that we focused on in this book, from start to finish, was how we could meet the needs of firefighters in all types of departments. We looked for alternative testing methods and fitness equipment for departments without a health and safety budget. We also focused on ways to keep the goal setting and monitoring simple and straightforward, knowing that firefighters often don't have a lot of time. The book also takes into consideration the lifestyle and daily routine of a firefighter and how that relates to nutritional recommendations.

In order to help firefighters develop the knowledge, skills, and abilities (KSAs) involved in designing a fitness program, the book utilized principles and research conducted by the American College of Sports Medicine (ACSM), the National Strength and Conditioning Association (NSCA), and the American Council on Exercise (ACE). KSAs crucial to achieving healthy and fit firefighters are:

- knowledge of the increased health risks associated with firefighting
- baseline assessment of physical condition and health risk status
- development of a plan using goal-setting techniques to improve the health risk factors
- the ability to mentally focus on training objectives
- cardiovascular conditioning, both aerobic and anaerobic
- total body muscular strength training
- core body strength
- balance training
- proper nutritional habits

No prerequisites or prior knowledge of fitness principles are needed to use this book. Firefighters and emergency service personnel who have an interest in improving their own health and fitness will find this book ideally suited to meet their needs.

ORGANIZATION OF THIS BOOK

The book is designed in a sequential format with each chapter building upon the knowledge and skills developed in the previous chapter(s).

The book is best used in the order presented. It is important to understand the concepts outlined in goal setting before embarking on a fitness regime. The book also provides some helpful charts and worksheets. Readers can use these to establish their goals, track nutrition, or monitor exercises or fitness routines.

- **Chapter One:** covers the physical and mental challenges inherent in firefighting, and the relationship between a firefighter's fitness level and the likelihood of cardiovascular disease and injury. In particular, the dramatic effect that increased fitness levels have on reducing line-of-duty deaths and injuries is presented along with the role that stress plays in firefighter health. The chapter includes the fire service's three-part response to these challenges by outlining the Wellness-Fitness Initiative, NFPA standards, and Life Safety Initiatives.

- **Chapter Two:** covers the four success principles of effective fitness program design. Goal setting, learning fitness principles, program planning, and feedback are defined and the function that each plays in effective fitness program development is shown.

- **Chapter Three:** outlines the essential components of fitness program design. A step-by-step process is presented that includes health screening, biometric testing, nutrition concepts, training principles, and mental focusing abilities.

- **Chapter Four:** introduces the concept of periodization, which allows firefighters to maximize results by scheduling their training in a progressive manner. Three different periodization models are presented, which allows firefighters to add variety to their training routines and prevents overtraining. The treatment of injuries and overtraining conditions is also addressed.

- **Chapter Five:** focuses on evaluating and changing a fire department's culture. The influence of culture on each firefighter's health is explored and departmental and individual change strategies detailed. The chapter also covers equipment selection and maintenance guidelines.

There are four appendices. Appendix A is a pictorial representation and description of basic weight training exercises. Appendix B contains medical screening and performance charts that allow firefighters to determine their risk factors and track their programs. Appendix C has equipment purchasing and maintenance checklists, and Appendix D is a listing of organizational resources and scientific references.

FEATURES

- **Practical Advice** for introducing change within the department, as well as guidance on equipment selection and maintenance guidelines are provided for the firefighter interested in developing a fitness program within his or her department.

- **Goal-Setting and Performance Planning Charts** allow firefighters to set learning and practice goals and detail how feedback will be received as their program progresses.

- **Case Studies** included in each chapter illustrates how firefighters and firefighter candidates can put exercises programs into practice

- **Resistance Training Exercises** are listed with an explanation of how each exercise relates to specific firefighter duties. Ideal and alternate exercises are listed to fit any department's budget and equipment availability.
- **Periodization Models and Program Design Examples** allow firefighters and firefighter candidates to add variety to their training programs.
- **Performance Points and Firefighter Fitness Facts** highlight expert advice on training and provide information on how a firefighter's fitness level affects his or her job performance.
- **Meets Recommended Guidelines** All recommended exercises, programs, and testing protocols are compatible with the Wellness-Fitness Initiative, NFPA 1583, and Firefighter Life Safety Initiatives.

- **Guidelines for Customizing Fitness Programs** address health risk factors, including low back injuries.

SUPPLEMENTAL PACKAGE

An **e.resource CD** available to instructors includes many helpful tools and resources:

- Answers to Review Questions
- Lesson Plans
- PowerPoint Presentations
- Chapter Quizzes
- Electronic versions of the screening and performance charts.

(Order#: 1-4283-6149-9)

Al Wasser is the Fitness Coordinator at Red Rocks Community College in Lakewood, Colorado. He has a Master's degree from Colorado State University and is an American Council on Exercise Gold certified personal trainer. He is also a Certified Strength and Conditioning Specialist (C.S.C.S.) from the National Strength and Conditioning Association. Al is coauthor of *Mastering the CPAT: A Comprehensive Guide*.

Andrea A. Walter is a freelance writer and editor specializing in fire and emergency service topics and a volunteer firefighter with the Sterling Volunteer Fire Company in Sterling, Virginia. She most recently worked as a firefighter/technician with the Metropolitan Washington Airports Authority at the Washington Dulles International Airport. She is a life member and former officer of the Sterling Volunteer Rescue Squad in Sterling, Virginia. Walter has been active in the fire and emergency services community for two decades. She has worked for the International Association of Fire Chiefs and has assisted with a variety of projects with the United States Fire Administration, the Federal Emergency Management Agency, Women in the Fire Service, and the National Volunteer Fire Council. Walter has been active with Delmar Cengage Learning for more than a decade, and serves as lead author for The Firefighter's Handbook; she is also co-author and content editor for The First Responder Handbook: Fire Service Edition, The First Responder Handbook: Law Enforcement Edition, Exam Preparation: Firefighter I and II, and Exam Preparation: Hazardous Material Awareness and Operations. Walter is a member of the National Fire Protection Association's Fire Fighter Professional Qualifications Committee.

Acknowledgements

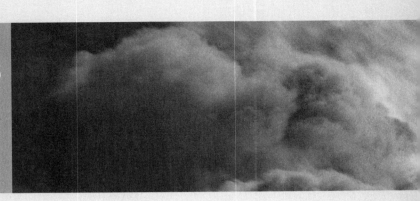

From Al: Special thanks to photographer Amy Glickson (www.pixlstudio.com).

From Andrea: I would like to thank the core revision author team from the *Firefighter's Handbook*, Third Edition, for their diligent focus on firefighter health and safety issues that caused me to see the need for this text.

The authors and publisher also wish to express their thanks for those reviewers who provided insight and guidance in the development of the manuscript:

Ben Andrews
Assistant Chief
Clallam County Fire District #3, WA

Rose Argo
Instructor, Fire Technology
Santa Ana College, CA

Debbie Birsh
Instructor, Recruit Firefighter Program
Connecticut Fire Academy, CT

Tony Calorel
Senior Instructor
Burlington County Emergency Services Training Center, NJ

Steve Malley
Department Chair, Public Safety Professions
Weatherford College, TX

George E. Petrovay
Instructor, Fire and Emergency Services
Hocking College, OH

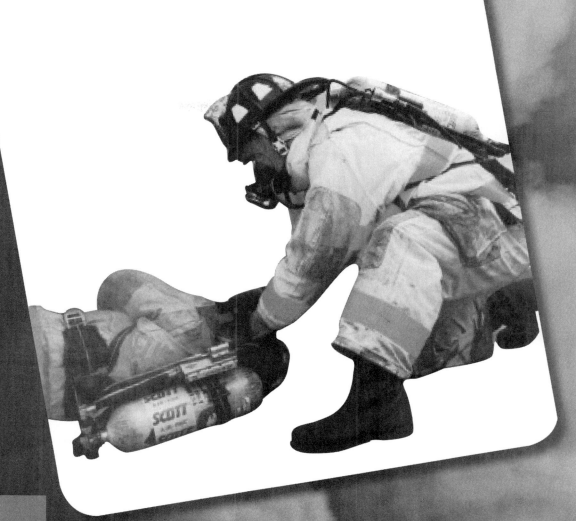

1

Health and Fitness of Firefighters

OBJECTIVES

Upon completion of this chapter, the firefighter will be able to

- Learn how fitness can reduce the risk of a heart attack
- Understand how cortisol impacts the body's immune system
- List and explain the five major topics of the Wellness-Fitness Initiative (WFI)
- Compare line-of-duty deaths (LODD) for firefighters with non-firefighting occupations

- List and contrast the effects of short-term and long-term stress exposure
- Explain how fitness and wellness help lessen the effects of stress
- Identify the factors contributing to line-of-duty (LODD) deaths for firefighters
- Learn how organizational culture can influence a firefighter's fitness level

PHYSICAL AND MENTAL CHALLENGES OF FIREFIGHTING

"When a man becomes a fireman his greatest act of bravery has been accomplished. What he does after that is all in the line of duty."
—Chief Edward Croker, FDNY, 1908

Firefighting is one of the most physically and mentally challenging jobs in North America.[1] Firefighter shift work requires long hours on duty, probable sleep deprivation, and intense physical efforts. Most duties are performed while wearing about 50 pounds of personal protective equipment, sometimes for prolonged periods. Stress levels are increased by over-exertion, the rising high-heat atmosphere, dense smoke exposure, reactions to alarm bells, exposure to tragedy, and overall mental demands of the job, **Figure 1-1**. Perhaps the most stressful demand is the very fast transition between being sedentary for long periods and sudden high levels of exertion or activity. A firefighter can go from sleeping in a bed to entering a fire in a matter of minutes. No exercise physiologist would advise a person to work at 100 percent effort without warming up. All of these factors create unique challenges for firefighters not encountered in other occupations.

One of the purposes of this text is to show firefighters the critical role fitness plays in the performance of duties, a firefighting career, and personal well-being both on and off the job. Another purpose of the text is to show firefighters strategies for defining and achieving fitness goals. It is not enough to show firefighters where the importance of fitness lies on the "map"; it is equally important to help them plan a route to get there.

INJURY AND MORBIDITY RATES OF FIREFIGHTERS

Firefighters have one of the nation's highest occupational injury and death rates. In addition, firefighters experience greater incidences of digestive, immune system, and cardiovascular disease than the general population.[2]

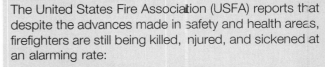

FIREFIGHTER FITNESS FACTS

The United States Fire Association (USFA) reports that despite the advances made in safety and health areas, firefighters are still being killed, injured, and sickened at an alarming rate:

- Firefighter **line-of-duty deaths (LODD)** and injuries occur at a rate one and one-half times those of police officers.
- Fatal heart attacks are the leading cause of LODD.
- According to the National Fire Protection Association, 80,100 firefighters were injured in the line of duty in 2005, an increase of 5.6 percent from 2004.
- A 2007 study found that the risk of a heart-related death while performing firefighting activities was up to one hundred times higher than the risk encountered when performing non-firefighter duties.[3]

ANALYSIS OF FIREFIGHTER INJURIES AND LINE OF DUTY DEATHS

Researchers believe that poor fitness and health levels (such as being overweight and in poor physical condition), combined with exposure to high and prolonged stress levels, may increase a firefighter's risk of dying from heart disease.

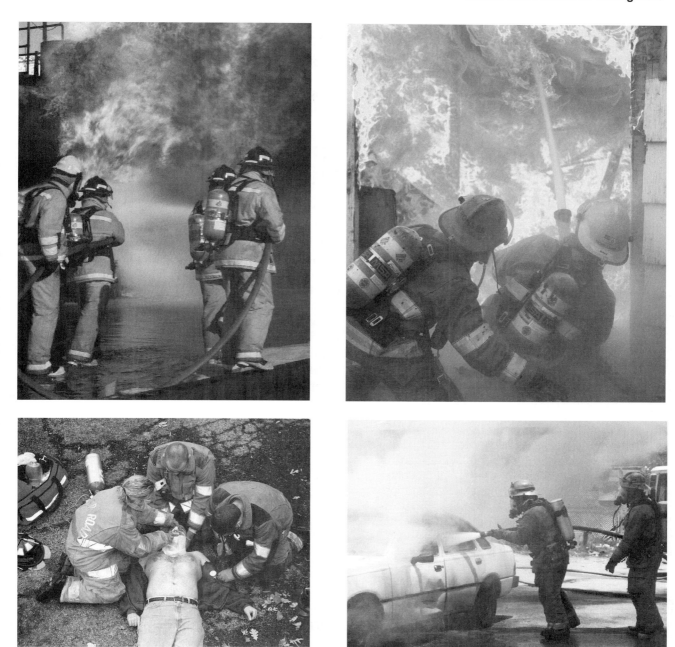

FIGURE 1-1 The physical demands of firefighting require firefighters to have a high fitness level.

Fitness and Health Levels

Researchers examining six years of firefighter line-of-duty-deaths (LODD) found that cardiovascular disease contributed to 53.3 percent of the fatalities, see **Figure 1-2** on the following page. Cardiovascular disease results in a restricted blood flow and a decrease in oxygen available to flow to the muscles. The rapid transition from rest or sleep to maximum

effort and the high demand for oxygen during firefighting activities coupled with this restricted blood flow increases the risk of a heart attack. Other factors contributing to LODD are personal protective equipment (19.41 percent) and human error (19.1 percent).

The study was conducted using data compiled over a six-year period (2000 to 2005) from four sources: the National Fire Protection Association (NFPA), the

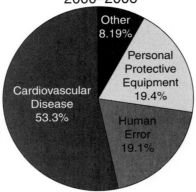

Firefighter Line-of-Duty-Deaths
2000–2006

FIGURE 1-2   Firefighter Line-of-Duty-Deaths 2000–2006.

National Institute for Occupational Safety and Health (NIOSH), the United States Fire Association (USFA), and the International Association of Fire Fighters (IAFF).[4]

FIREFIGHTER FITNESS FACTS

The Internet provides firefighters with a myriad of resources to research and learn about firefighter injuries and LODD. There are many websites and organizations devoted to finding out the facts about firefighter injuries and LODD and providing these facts and lessons learned to other firefighters in the hopes of avoiding history repeating itself. Firefighters should make it a part of their jobs to read these case studies and reports and try to learn from these incidents.

Stress Levels

When the body is in a stressful situation, it adapts with the fight-or-flight response. This is achieved with the release of adrenaline and cortisol from the adrenal glands. **Cortisol**, sometimes called "the stress hormone," is a hormone produced by the adrenal glands that helps regulate blood pressure and cardiovascular function, as well as the metabolism and breakdown of proteins, carbohydrates, and fats. Cortisol secretion increases in response to physical and psychological stress. At normal levels, cortisol helps the body react to stress appropriately and provides sources of energy. Positive adaptations to normal stress include increased concentration, ability to focus on the stressor, increased blood flow to the muscles, and heightened awareness. When stress exposure is prolonged or frequent, high levels of cortisol in the bloodstream have been shown to diminish cognitive performance, suppress thyroid function, decrease bone density, decrease muscle tissue, increase blood pressure, and increase abdominal fat. These negative effects can lead to increased risk of heart attack and stroke.[5]

THE ROLE OF FITNESS IN REDUCING FIREFIGHTER INJURIES AND LODD

Will LODD and injuries be reduced or eliminated if fitness levels are improved? Many studies have shown that as fitness levels go up, heart attack risk decreases. A worldwide study of 30,000 people in 52 countries found that the majority of heart attacks may be predicted by three measurable factors: cigarette smoking, high cholesterol levels, and lack of exercise. The study also identified three behaviors that are protective against heart attacks: daily consumption of fruits and vegetables, regular physical exercise, and moderate alcohol consumption (three times per week), **Figure 1-3**.[6]

The Institute for Aerobics Research in Dallas, Texas, performed an eight-year study of more than 13,000 men and women. Researchers concluded that the higher an individual's fitness level, the lower the subsequent death rate from heart attack and cancer.[7]

A University of Arkansas research team designed a three-month conditioning program for firefighters. The goal was to determine if an exercise program combined with information about nutrition and stress reduction could reduce the incidence of stress in firefighters. "In just five weeks of the pilot project, we saw dramatic improvements in endurance and stamina," said Barry Brown, a university professor of exercise science.[8]

The most prominent study on the influence of fitness on heart disease risk comes from the American Heart Association. The 2007 data update clearly indicates that increases in fitness levels will result in decreases in injuries and cardiovascular stress.[9]

FIRE SERVICE HEALTH AND FITNESS INITIATIVES

In reaction to the increased health risks faced by firefighters, the fire and emergency service community has developed three initiatives: The Joint Labor Management Wellness-Fitness Initiative, NFPA Standards, and Firefighter Life Safety Initiatives.

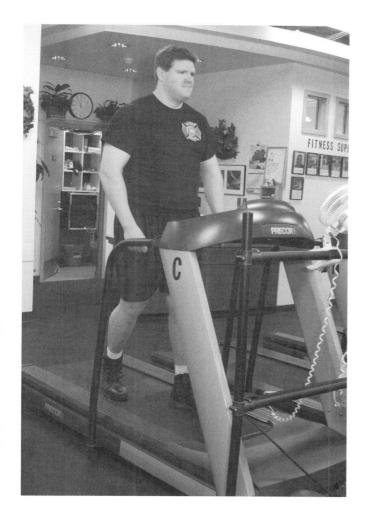

FIGURE 1-3 Regular exercise will lower your heart disease risk.

The Joint Labor and Management Wellness-Fitness Initiative (WFI)

In 1996, the **International Association of Fire Chiefs (IAFC)** and the **International Association of Fire Fighters (IAFF)** came together to write and implement the Joint Labor and Management Wellness-Fitness Initiative (WFI). The IAFC represents over 12,000 fire chiefs and fire department chief officers, and the IAFF represents over 230,000 professional firefighters and emergency personnel. The goal of the WFI is to promote wellness and fitness as a job qualification and a lifestyle, to improve the quality of life, and to prolong a high quality career and life for all firefighters.

To accomplish these goals, the WFI focuses on five topics of importance: medical evaluation, fitness testing and exercise, rehabilitation, behavioral health promotion, and data collection.

Medical Evaluation. Management and Labor shall support the provision of the comprehensive mandatory annual medical exams by the Fire Department as a component of the Wellness-Fitness Program. All uniformed personnel should have a yearly exam administered by a physician who is familiar with NFPA standard 1582 to determine if the firefighter is physically capable of performing his or her duties, **Figure 1-4**. NFPA standard 1582 requires that candidates meet all the medical requirements set forth in this document regardless of how well they do on the rest of the recruiting process.

Fitness Testing and Exercise. Management and Labor shall work together to provide workout scheduling, resource support, and/or access to resources on duty to support an individualized fitness program. All fire department members should have a yearly fitness assessment. The **Candidate Physical Ability Test (CPAT)** was created through the WFI to evaluate a new candidate's readiness to meet the high physical demands of firefighting, **Figure 1-5** on page 7. Some fire departments use the CPAT, or some form of the CPAT, to measure physical abilities of firefighters on a recurring basis, not just at their entry into the fire department.

Rehabilitation. Management and labor shall work together to provide a progressive individualized injury/fitness/medical rehabilitation of any affected uniformed personnel to a safe return to duty status. After an injury or illness a firefighter must be rehabilitated and released by a physician before returning to duty.

Behaviorial Health Promotion. Management and Labor shall support the provision of a behavioral health plan which may be delivered either through internal or external sources, based on specific elements. Many departments offer **Employee Assistance Programs** (counseling services), and **Critical Incident Stress Debriefing Programs** (informal counseling programs to assist after traumatic incidents), **Figure 1-6** on page 7.

Data Collection. The data component of the WFI includes the storage and analysis of detailed case information related to medical condition (exam/laboratory data), fitness, rehabilitation, and behavioral health. Information is collected in a uniform and consistent manner and then uploaded into the International Wellness-Fitness Database. All personal health data collected is kept confidential.

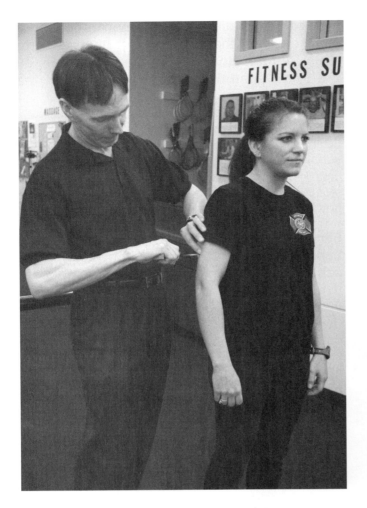
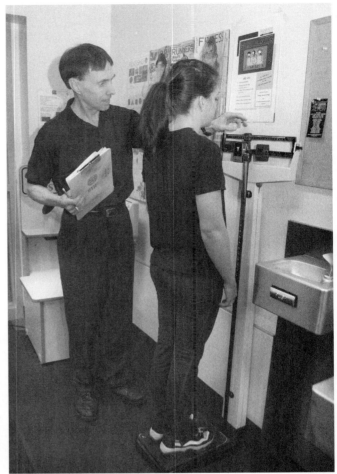
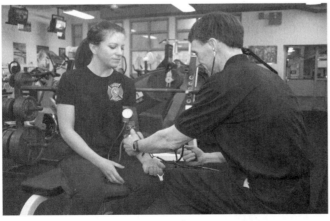
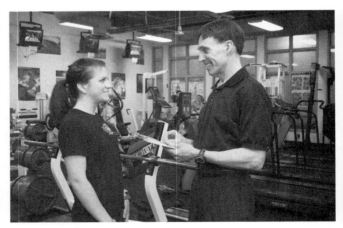

FIGURE 1-4   Maximizing each firefighter's fitness and health is the goal of the WFI.

NFPA Standards

The **National Fire Protection Association (NFPA)** creates a wide variety of consensus-based standards for fire departments on topics from fire apparatus to health and safety. There are three key NFPA standards that relate to the discussion of fitness programs for firefighters.

NFPA 1500.   NFPA 1500, *Standard on Fire Department Occupational Safety and Health Program*, is a broad-reaching standard that focuses on a variety of programs and issues that fire departments can focus on to improve health and safety for members. This standard advocates the use of a physical fitness program in fire departments.

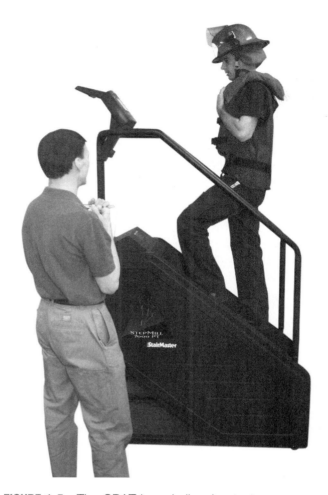

FIGURE 1-5 The CPAT is a challenging test.

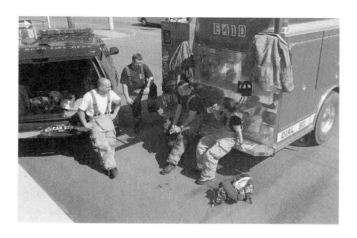

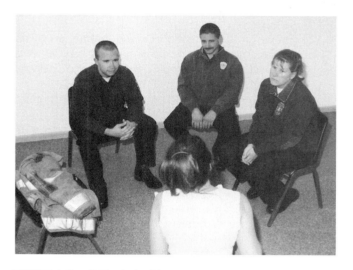

FIGURE 1-6 Critical incident stress-management sessions are crucial for managing stress.

NFPA 1582. NFPA 1582, *Standard on Medical Requirements for Fire Fighters and Information for Fire Department Physicians*, promotes annual medical examinations for firefighters.

NFPA 1583. Perhaps the most relevant to our discussion on fitness programs is NFPA 1583, *Standard on Health-Related Fitness Programs for Fire Fighters*. This standard contains information for fire departments to put fitness programs in place, and presents the minimum requirements for programs to be effective for firefighters. This standard was designed to work with the other NFPA standards listed above and also to work in tandem with the IAFF/IAFC Wellness-Fitness Initiative. The fitness discussions and recommendations in this text are aligned with the recommendations set forth in NFPA 1583.

Firefighter Safety Initiatives

In 2004, the USFA and the National Fallen Firefighters Foundation (NFFF) hosted a summit to discuss firefighter death and injury trends. From that meeting, sixteen Firefighter Life Safety Initiatives were developed to help reach a stated goal of reducing firefighter fatalities by 50 percent in ten years.

These studies and initiatives, as well as many others, make it very clear that there is a dramatic relationship between fitness and health and firefighter injuries and LODD. While it is understood that firefighting can be a demanding and sometimes dangerous job, research and past experience is showing us that there are steps we can take to help avoid injuries and LODD.

CASE STUDY: DEVELOPING A WELLNESS AND FITNESS CULTURE

Culture is the collection of values, norms, legends, and beliefs that differentiate one group from another. Most people in business and other organizations would say that culture is "the way things are done around here." If an organization's culture is not in alignment with its strategy, the organization will not be successful. According to Dr. Rick Bellingham, CEO and founder of the strategic management firm Jobility, "It doesn't matter if you have the best goals and strategy ever conceived, if the culture doesn't support them, and in fact resists them, you're already poised for failure."

16 FIREFIGHTER LIFE SAFETY INITIATIVES

1. Define and advocate the need for a cultural change within the fire service relating to safety; incorporating leadership, management, supervision, accountability, and personal responsibility.
2. Enhance the personal and organizational accountability for health and safety throughout the fire service.
3. Focus greater attention on the integration of risk management with incident management at all levels, including strategic, tactical, and planning responsibilities.
4. All firefighters must be empowered to stop unsafe practices.
5. Develop and implement national standards for training, qualifications, and certification (including regular recertification) that are equally applicable to all firefighters based on the duties they are expected to perform.
6. Develop and implement national medical and physical fitness standards that are equally applicable to all firefighters, based on the duties they are expected to perform.
7. Create a national research agenda and data collection system that relates to the initiatives.
8. Utilize available technology wherever it can produce higher levels of health and safety.
9. Thoroughly investigate all firefighter fatalities, injuries, and near misses.
10. Grant programs should support the implementation of safe practices and/or mandate safe practices as an eligibility requirement.
11. National standards for emergency response policies and procedures should be developed and championed.
12. National protocols for response to violent incidents should be developed and championed.
13. Firefighters and their families must have access to counseling and psychological support.
14. Public education must receive more resources and be championed as a critical fire and life safety program.
15. Advocacy must be strengthened for the enforcement of codes and the installation of home fire sprinklers.
16. Safety must be a primary consideration in the design of apparatus and equipment.

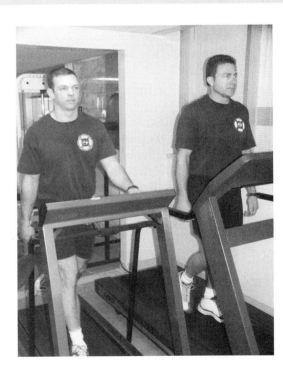

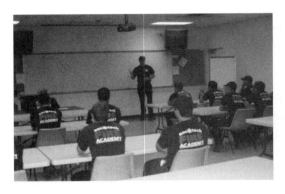

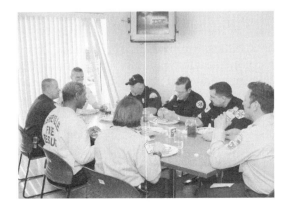

FIGURE 1-7   A supportive culture that includes good nutrition, exercise, and education will enhance a firefighter's health.

Most organizations have incongruencies or gaps between what is said to be important and what the reality is. From an employee point of view, workplace culture makes the difference in achieving health, productivity, and innovation. It's easy to see how a negative, stress-filled environment can cause illness and distress. The influence of a negative or incongruent culture is shown in two studies that revealed that heart attacks are 2.6 times more frequent among firefighters of lower fitness levels as compared with firefighters who were more physically fit. Back injuries were seven times greater among the former group.[10,11]

The opposite is also true: a supportive, congruent environment enhances productivity and can create a healthy employee, **Figure 1-7**. A firefighter culture that promotes healthy nutrition, provides exercise time and facilities, and offers stress-management training will increase a firefighter's fitness level and ability to tolerate the stresses involved in the job.

This case study presented an overview of organizational culture and the dramatic influence that it has on the health of an individual. In subsequent chapters, we will examine the process of developing a culture that supports each firefighter's fitness and health.

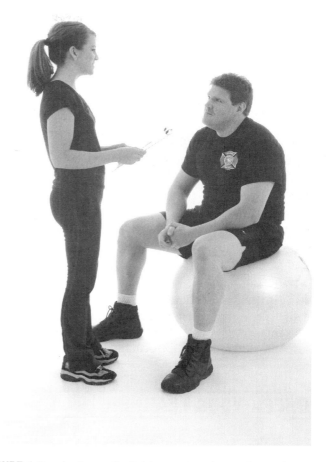

FIGURE 1-8 Just one firefighter can make an impact on a fire department's culture.

NOTES

It is important to realize that, as a firefighter, you can affect the culture of an organization. Making time every day to exercise, on duty and off duty, demonstrates to others around you the importance and value of fitness. The more shift members that catch on to this, the more people will exercise and improve their fitness levels. It can start with just one firefighter, **Figure 1-8**.

CHAPTER SUMMARY

Firefighters have one of the nation's highest occupational injury and death rates. Fatal heart attacks are the leading cause of line-of-duty deaths (LODD) and injuries occur at a much higher rate when compared to other occupations. A firefighter's life expectancy is significantly shorter (by about 10 years) than the general population. Firefighters also experience greater incidences of digestive, immune system, and cardiovascular disease than the general population. In 2005, the injury rate for firefighters increased by 5.6 percent over 2004 totals.

Researchers believe that being overweight and in poor physical condition combined with exposure to high and prolonged stress increases a firefighter's risk of dying from heart disease. Cortisol, a hormone, is produced by the adrenal glands in response to physical and psychological stress. At normal levels, cortisol helps the body react to stress appropriately and provides sources of energy. When stress exposure is prolonged or frequent, high levels of cortisol in the bloodstream have been shown to produce negative effects that can lead to increased risk of heart attack and stroke.

In an effort to promote wellness and fitness among firefighters and to increase the quality of life for all fire department members, the International Association of Chiefs (IAFC) and the International Association of Firefighters (IAFF) developed the Joint Labor Management Wellness-Fitness Initiative. The WFI consists of five specific areas: medical evaluation, fitness testing and exercise, rehabilitation, behavioral health promotion, and data collection.

Culture has a dramatic influence on the fitness and wellness levels of firefighters. Congruency between an organization's values and reality will enhance fit- ness levels, while incongruencies will reduce a firefighter's ability to tolerate job-related stress.

KEY TERMS

Candidates Physical Ability Test (CPAT)   An eight-event physical test that measures a candidate's ability to perform firefighting tasks

Cortisol   A hormone secreted by the adrenal glands in response to stressful situations

Critical Incident Stress Debriefing (CISD)   A formal gathering of incident responders to help diffuse and address stress from a given incident

Culture   The collection of values, norms, legends, and beliefs that differentiate one group from another

Employee Assistance Program (EAP)   A cost-effective, humanitarian, job-based strategy for helping employees whose personal problems are affecting their work performance

Firefighter Life Safety Initiatives   A sixteen-part program developed by the United States Fire Association (USFA) and National Fallen Firefighters Foundation (NFFF) designed to reduce firefighter fatalities by 50 percent within ten years

Joint Labor and Management Wellness-Fitness Initiative (WFI)   A five-part initiative designed by the fire chiefs and firefighters' unions to address the rising number of firefighter deaths and injuries

Line-of-duty deaths (LODD)   Fatalities resulting from performing firefighting tasks

National Fire Protection Association (NFPA)   A nonprofit membership organization that uses a consensus process to develop model fire prevention codes and firefighting training standards

CHECK YOUR LEARNING

1. Prolonged exposure to cortisol
   a. increases concentration ability.
   b. increases the risk of heart disease.
   c. stabilizes blood pressure.
   d. decreases abdominal fat.
2. The goal of the Joint Labor Management Wellness-Fitness Initiative is to
   a. decrease workers' compensation claims.
   b. promote fitness, to improve the quality of life, and prolong a quality career for all firefighters.
   c. find the toughest, strongest men in the community.
   d. discipline those that can't keep up the high physical standards of firefighting.
3. What percentage of LODD is attributed to cardiovascular disease?
   a. 35%
   b. 18%
   c. 53%
   d. 78%
4. All of the following are contributing factors to LODD except
   a. personal protective equipment.
   b. human error.

   c. fitness and wellness.
   d. age.
5. The leading cause/s of LODD is/are
   a. injuries.
   b. heart attacks.
   c. personal protective equipment.
   d. lack of training.
6. Cortisol's function is to
   a. help regulate blood pressure and cardiovascular function.
   b. increase stress levels.
   c. increase concentration ability.
   d. heighten awareness levels.
   e. do all of the above.
7. According to the National Fire Protection Association, firefighter injuries for 2005 changed by what percent compared with 2004?
   a. decreased by 2.9%
   b. increased by 10.2%
   c. remained about the same
   d. increased by 5.6%
8. The Candidates Physical Abilities Test (CPAT) was designed to
   a. determine if a firefighter has recovered sufficiently from an injury.

b. evaluate a candidate's readiness to meet the physical demands of firefighting.

c. detect any changes in health and ability of firefighters.

d. decrease workers' compensation claims.

9. Normal stress levels are associated with all of the following except

a. increased awareness of surroundings.

b. increased blood flow to the muscles.

c. ability to focus on the stressor.

d. anxiety.

10. All of the following are part of the Wellness-Fitness Initiative except

a. data collection.

b. fitness testing and exercise.

c. body fat composition.

d. behavioral health promotion.

11. Incongruencies in organizational culture produce

a. alignments with strategy.

b. increased productivity.

c. healthy employees.

d. decreased stress levels.

e. increased stress levels.

REFERENCES

1. International Association of Firefighters, AFL-CIO, CLC. (1999). *The Fire Service Joint Labor Management Wellness-Fitness Initiative*. (Washington, DC: Author).

2. American Council on Exercise. (2003). ACE Personal Trainer Manual (3d ed). (San Diego, CA: Author).

3. Kales, S.N.; Soteriades, E.S.; Christophi, C.A.; and Christiani, D.C. "Emergency duties and deaths from Heart Disease among Firefighters in the United States" *New England Journal of Medicine*, vol. 356, number 12, (March 22, 2007): 1207–1215.

4. Smith, S. "Health and Fitness Leading Contributors to Firefighter Line-of-Duty Deaths" *Responder Safety*, (December 7, 2006).

5. Scott, E. "Cortisol and Stress: How to Stay Healthy" About.com: Stress Management. (2006).

6. INTERHEART STUDY, *The Lancet* (2004; 364:9438, 937–52) (September 11, 2004).

7. "Cardiorespiratory Fitness as a Predictor of Cardiovascular events" *American Journal of Epidemiology*, volume 165, issue 12: (June, 15, 2007).

8. University of Arkansas *Research Frontiers*, (Spring 2005).

9. American Heart Association. (2007). Heart Disease and Stroke Statistics-2007 Update. (Dallas, TX: American Heart Association).

10. Cady, L.D.; Bischoff, D.P.; O'Connel, E. R.; Thomas, P.C.; and Allen, J.H. "Strength and Fitness and subsequent back injuries in firefighters" *Journal of Occupational Medicine*. 24 (1979): 269–272.

11. Cady, Lee D.; Thomas, P.; and Karwasky, R. "Program for increasing health and physical fitness of five fighters" *Journal of Occupational Medicine*. 27 (2) (February 1985): 110–114.

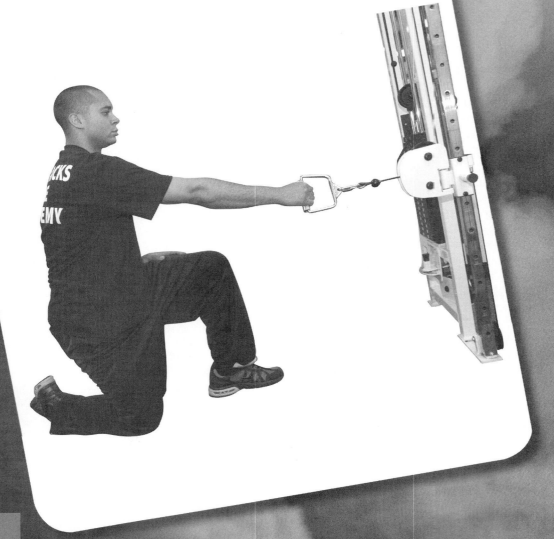

2

The Four Success Principles

Upon completion of this chapter, the firefighter will be able to

- List and explain the four principles of designing a successful fitness program
- List three reasons why goal setting is important
- Define the SMART goal-setting technique
- Define what a learning point is and give two examples

- Define and give an example of overlearning
- Explain the importance of planning in developing a successful program
- List five guidelines associated with feedback

INTRODUCTION

Most successful fitness programs consist of four principles: goal setting, skill learning, program planning, and receiving feedback.[1] These principles provide a framework by which you can acquire the knowledge, skills, and abilities necessary for designing a successful fitness program. Each principle is described in this chapter with guidelines and examples of how to use them to develop your training program.

PRINCIPLE ONE: SETTING GOALS

"Whatever the mind of man can conceive and believe it can achieve."

—From the classic *Think and Grow Rich* by Napoleon Hill

Why Goal Setting is Important

Goal setting is the foundation upon which you will design your training program. It will guide what you do, when you will do it, and at what intensity. When combined with the other success principles, it will allow you to gauge the effectiveness of your training and help you to know when to make adjustments or take a rest day. As you accomplish your goals, you will train with confidence, vision, and enthusiasm. Train without setting goals and you will lack direction, purpose, mental focus, and most of all, results.

The fire service is full of great examples of goal setters who accomplish a wide variety of tasks. We all know someone in our department who set a goal of completing college or getting a promotion, made a plan, and stuck to it until they accomplished what they set out to do. Even the way in which we deal with emergency situations is often goal oriented. Obviously, a firefighter's task is to put out the fire, but we have a whole host of goals involved in the fireground effort for the many teams assigned to work there such as accomplishing a primary search, laddering a building, and ventilating a roof. Sometimes a discussion of goal setting seems foreign to firefighters before they realize that goal setting is a part of everyday life in the fire service, **Figure 2-1**. It is how we can get the job done, whether it be extinguishing a fire or improving our fitness levels.

Your behavior and intentions are regulated by the goals you have set.[2] The quality of your training is dependent on your appraisal of what is to be done, how well you are prepared to do it, and whether you think it can or cannot be done. When you clearly know what you want and are determined to reach it, your goals will allow you to focus your energy on achieving the desired outcome.

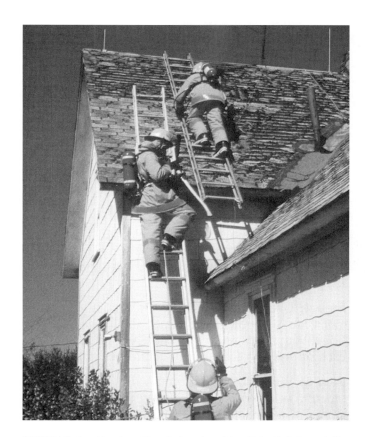

FIGURE 2-1   Goal setting is involved in all firefighting skills.

Goal-Setting Guidelines

Step 1: Define your training goals by using the **SMART** technique:

S-Specific. Specific goals lead to higher levels of achievement than generalized goals or the setting of no goals at all.

M-Measurable. You must be able to measure progress as you go along. If your goals are not measurable, you won't know where you stand on the road to your goal.

A-Attainable. You must believe that the goal is possible. Your subconscious will not commit to an unattainable goal.

R-Realistic. Realistic, challenging goals result in higher levels of performance than do no goals or generalized goals such as "Do your best." If the goal is too easy, you will lose interest and commitment. Setting your goals just above your past level of performance will increase your motivation.

T-Time-based. You must develop a timeline for each of your goals. This will allow you to know exactly where you should be at any specific point in time. List exact dates and times, and include a date for final completion of the goal.

Step 2: Goals should be set by you and *written down*. By consciously setting and writing down your goals, you will subconsciously commit to them.

Step 3: Your initial goals should be *simple and achievable*. Accomplishing these small goals will build the foundation necessary for setting more challenging goals later on.

Step 4: Under each goal make a list of *objectives:* What are you going to do each day, each week, to bring you closer to your goal? As you accomplish each of these objectives your confidence will grow.

Step 5: Write down how you will *reward yourself* when you achieve a goal. Draw up a goal and rewards contract with your friends, relatives, shift mates, or shift commander.

Step 6: *Sign* your written goal plan. You will then have committed yourself to take action.

Step 7: *Evaluate* your goals often. You will need to adjust any unmet goals.

PRINCIPLE TWO: LEARNING FITNESS PRINCIPLES

I hear and I forget
I see and I remember
I do and I understand

—Confucius

Why Learning is Important

Training without a knowledge of proper exercise techniques and program design principles leads to guesswork, wasted effort, injury, and frustration. These skills need to be developed prior to starting your training program.

Learning physical skills requires viewing and practicing proper technique, **Figure 2-2.** By viewing exercise techniques, we form ideas of how physical behaviors are performed and the effects they produce.

Repeating the essential movements involved in each exercise will provide your body with the internal cues that regulate motor performance. As you execute each movement with perfect technique, over time the internal cues leading to errors are eliminated and those associated with smooth and precise performance are retained.

Nonphysical components of fitness, such as mental, nutritional, and program design principles are learned through comprehending the concepts and then understanding why they are important in achieving fitness goals.

There are three different outcomes that result from your learning sessions:

1. **Positive outcome**: the learning situation results in better performance.
2. **Negative outcome**: the learning situation results in poorer performance.

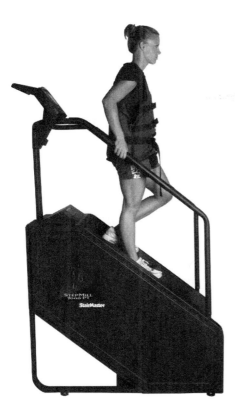

FIGURE 2-2 Learning good technique helps to develop new skills.

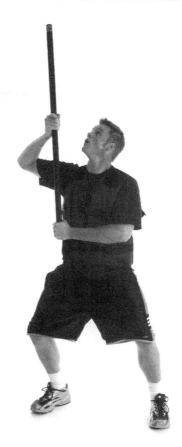

FIGURE 2-3 Watch for the learning points for each fire-fighter skill and exercise.

3. Neutral outcome: the learning situation has no effect on performance.

Use the following guidelines to maximize positive outcomes from learning situations.

Learning Guidelines

a. Watch for **learning points**, **Figure 2-3** in each exercise. Learning points are key behaviors or techniques that lead to success in each exercise. For instance, keeping the chest out and the eyes looking straight forward are two key learning points for the squat exercise.

b. Learn the basics first. Add the more complicated techniques after you have mastered the basics.

c. **Overlearning** entails putting in extra practice on skills you have already mastered.[4] Overlearning makes your performance more reflexive, or automatic, and enhances your ability to train in a fatigued state, see **Figure 2-4** on the next page. This increased level of fitness increases your firefighting endurance capacity, which in turn allows you to overlearn firefighting techniques.

d. Observing and practicing proper exercise technique is the best way to learn exercises. Try to view several examples of instances that do and do not represent the concepts being taught. The National Strength and Conditioning Association produces several exercise DVDs that demonstrate both proper and improper exercise technique.

e. When learning nonphysical fitness principles, make sure you understand the concept and the role it plays in enhancing fitness. Your subconscious will not commit to a concept that is not clear and purposeful.

PROMOTING FIREFIGHTER FITNESS

One Step at a Time

In the early stages of training, when you are trying to master the skills, a complex exercise such as walking lunges should be broken down into parts and learned progressively, one section at a time.

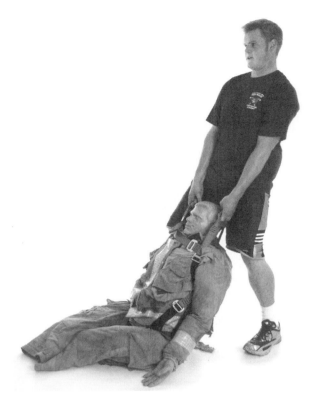

FIGURE 2-4   Overlearning a skill makes it more "reflexive," or automatic.

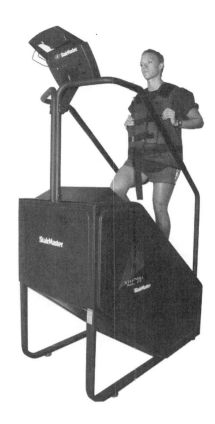

PRINCIPLE THREE: PLANNING YOUR PROGRAM

"It wasn't raining when Noah built the ark."
—Howard Ruff

Why planning is important

To achieve your fitness goals you must train correctly, follow an appropriate diet, get adequate rest, and effectively deal with stress. Many people have failed to see results because they followed programs they got from other people, magazines, or the Internet. Your program must be specific to your needs. A program that works for one individual may not work for another because people vary in their body types, ages, medical conditions, and so on. In order to make your own individualized program, you must carefully plan it to balance your health, fitness, and occupational goals, **Figure 2-5**.

Developing a plan will give direction to your training and allow you to focus on the task at hand. Using your goals as guidelines, planning will help you to develop a program that focuses on your unique needs and interests, **Figure 2-6**. If unanticipated conditions arise, planning will help you develop new goals.

Chapter 3 in this text has performance-planning charts that will guide you through the planning process.

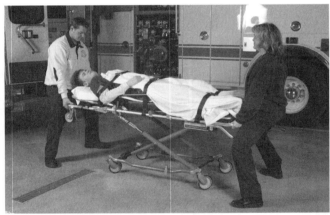

FIGURE 2-5   Exercising on the stepmill with a weighted vest builds the strength necessary for lifting victims.

Planning Guidelines

Use the following principles to plan out your fitness program:

a. Develop starting points for all your exercises by using the results from your biometric tests (see Chapter 3). This will provide you with baseline measures and allow you to set goals for the entire program.

b. Balance your program. Include a variety of cardiovascular conditioning activities (for example, walking, running, biking, and swimming), strength training, and flexibility exercises.

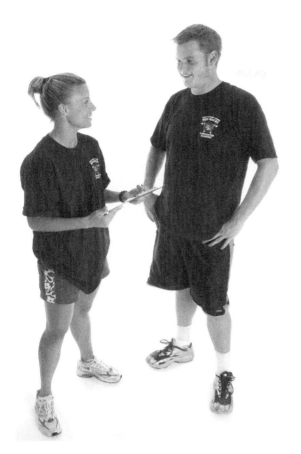

FIGURE 2-6 Guidance received from an experienced fire-fighter is invaluable for program planning.

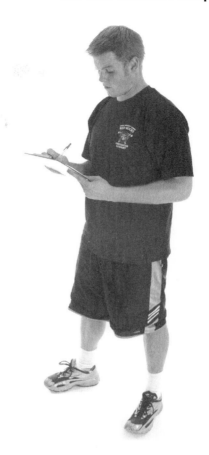

FIGURE 2-7 Evaluating your goals will keep you on track.

c. Develop a personalized plan based upon your specific needs.

d. Evaluate your goals often. Use the feedback from your training records to determine if your objectives are being met, **Figure 2-7**. Using a visual display of your training progress, such as a graph, is an excellent way of doing this. This will help you to redesign the program if necessary, adjust your training schedule, and reset your goals appropriately.

e. Schedule rest and recuperation periods in your plan. Chapter 4 has planning examples that show how to incorporate these into your schedule.

f. If you miss a week of training because of illness or injury, begin again where you left off. Don't skip ahead.

PRINCIPLE FOUR: FEEDBACK
Why Feedback is Important

Imagine competing in a sporting event without keeping score. Now imagine starting a training program and not having any idea of what exercises to do,

whether your form and technique are safe and efficient, or whether the nutritional plan you started is effective. You would be frustrated and your motivation would drop. When learning and implementing a new training program, **feedback**, or knowledge of results, is critical for both learning and motivation, see **Figure 2-8** on the following page.

Having clear goals is not enough. You must feel moment-by-moment that you are on your way toward reaching those goals. Feedback serves three purposes:

1. It conveys information to you about your performance.

2. It keeps your motivation high.

3. It allows you to set or modify your goals.

Feedback Guidelines

a. Feedback is neither good nor bad in itself. It is simply information that can be used to monitor and adjust your performance as needed.

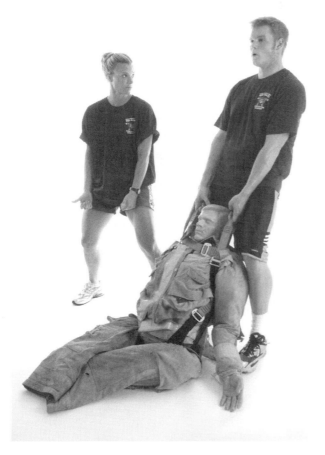

FIGURE 2-8 Good feedback is crucial when learning a firefighter skill.

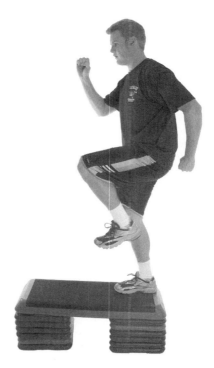

FIGURE 2-9 Developing kinesthetic awareness will help your exercise and firefighter performance.

e. Feedback from performance measures such as actual repetitions and sets completed, weights used, heart rate achieved, total exercise time, and nutritional records will allow you to pinpoint areas where improvement is needed.

b. The internal feedback from movements of the body allows you to make ongoing adjustments to keep on track or to get back on it. You know when movements have the right "feel" or your performance was "smooth." Known as **kinesthetic awareness**, this feel for one's performance is a key source of feedback when training, **Figure 2-9**.

c. External feedback should be provided immediately, as soon as possible after your workout. Videotaping your performance, a training partner or personal trainer, and other firefighters can provide this immediate feedback. Poor technique should be corrected straight away, to prevent injury.

d. Results from health screening and physical fitness tests will provide you with important feedback on your health-risk status and beginning physical condition levels.

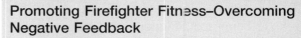

FIREFIGHTER FITNESS FACTS

Promoting Firefighter Fitness–Overcoming Negative Feedback

Our greatest glory is not in never falling, but in rising every time we fall

—Confucius

It is difficult to keep a positive attitude in the face of criticism or negative feedback. It is easy to lose confidence by focusing on errors and the perception that you are failing. Yet, it is what you decide to do with incoming information that has the biggest influence on your state of mind. What should you do when it seems that things are not going well? Michael Jordan said, in an advertisement, "I've failed over and over again in my life, and that is why I succeed." This quote by Jordan is also a reminder that challenge is the key to successful experiences. How the mind reacts is at least as important as the actual error itself.

CASE STUDIES

Using the Four Success Principles

Case Study One

Jennifer, a firefighter in a city fire department, was having trouble meeting her departmental physical fitness requirements. Stair climbing left her breathless and she could not complete the dummy (165 pound mannequin) drag test.

A physical checkup revealed that her cholesterol level was elevated (240 mg/dL) and that she was approximately 20 pounds overweight. Her doctor recommended that she contract the services of a personal trainer to develop an exercise and nutrition program. Jennifer set four goals after going through initial health screening and biometric fitness testing with a personal trainer:

Goal 1: Decrease her body fat percentage from 26 percent to 20 percent

Objective 1: Lose 0.5 percent of her body fat per week for twelve weeks.
Objective 2: Increase her meal frequency from two meals per day to six meals per day. (Jennifer will increase her meal frequency by one meal per day each week for a period of four weeks until she is up to six meals per day).
Objective 3: Increase her water intake to one gallon daily.

Goal 2: Increase her upper- and lower-body strength by 30 percent

Objective: A certified personal trainer will develop a strength training schedule for her.

Goal 3: Reduce her total cholesterol from 240 to 180. Increase her HDL or good cholesterol from 40 to 55

Objective 1: Enroll in a nutrition course offered by the local community college.
Objective 2: Have a blood panel test every two months.

Goal 4: Receive feedback on the effectiveness of her strength and cardiovascular training goals

Objective 1: Have biometric testing done initially and then every four weeks.

Objective 2: Keep detailed records on her training sessions.

Case study two: Art, a firefighter in a suburban fire and emergency service department, suffered a lower back injury while responding to an emergency call. His injury was diagnosed as a severe lower back strain caused by overtaxed back muscles. His physician said that this resulted from Art's being severely overweight (e.g., Art has a 40" waistline) and recommended that he begin an exercise and nutrition program. Art set three health and fitness goals:

Goal 1: Reduce his body weight from 240 to 200 pounds

Objective 1: Run up the stairs at the local high school three times per week.
Objective 2: Complete three high-intensity weight-training sessions each week.

Goal 2: Increase his protein intake

Objective 1: Drink three protein shakes per day.

Objective 2: Include 8 ounces of protein at each of his regular meals.

Goal 3: Start a fitness program

Objective 1: Read several exercise and fitness magazines.
Objective 2: Talk to other firefighters assigned to his station about their training techniques.

Case Study Questions:

1. How has Jennifer incorporated the four success principles in her training plan?
2. How well has Art incorporated the four success principles into his training plan?
3. Are the goals and objectives Jennifer set effective in helping her improve her fitness levels?
4. What other goals could Art set to help him improve his fitness levels?

CHAPTER SUMMARY

Successful fitness training programs consist of four key principles: goal setting, learning the skills, planning the program, and receiving feedback.

Setting goals using the SMART (specific, measurable, attainable, realistic, and time-oriented) technique will direct and guide your training. Training goals should be reevaluated and adjusted according to external feedback received from biometric testing and workout sessions, as well as internal feedback from repeated movements. To be effective, goals should be written down and signed, and you should reward yourself when you accomplish your goals.

When learning exercise techniques it is important to note key behaviors or learning points that lead to successful execution of each exercise. Maximize your learning by studying models that are similar to you in sex, body size, and so on. Overlearning involves practicing training skills far beyond the point of mastery. This increases one's endurance capability for firefighter tasks.

Planning your program will give focus and direction to your training. A properly planned program based upon your unique needs and capabilities will enhance your chances of achieving your goals.

Feedback provides information on your performance, keeps your motivation high, and allows you to set or modify goals. A key source of feedback is kinesthetic awareness that is generated from movements of the body while training. Feedback from training sessions should be received as soon as possible and broken down into specifics for each exercise, such as time spent, repetitions and sets completed, weight lifted, and intensity levels. Biometric measures are also useful feedback.

KEY TERMS

Active practice   Active practice provides as much experience as possible with an exercise or learning experience

Feedback   Specific information provided about a given performance

Goal setting   Goal setting is the foundation on which training is designed

Kinesthetic awareness   The ability to recognize when movements have the right "feel" or that performance was "smooth"

Learning point   Key behaviors or techniques that lead to successful execution of a movement

Overlearning   Practicing beyond the point of mastery for a given movement

Reflexive   Automatic, or without conscious control

SMART goal-setting technique   Setting goals that are specific, measurable, attainable, realistic, and time-oriented

CHECK YOUR LEARNING

1. Goal-setting principles include
   a. writing down your goals.
   b. listing objectives for each major goal.
   c. writing broad, unspecific goals.
   d. evaluating your goals often.
   e. a, b, and d.
2. The SMART goal setting technique includes
   a. time-oriented goals.
   b. extraordinary goals.
   c. do-your-best goals.
   d. non-specific goals.
3. The *most* effective way to learn a proper exercise technique is to
   a. try it yourself.
   b. talk to several gym members.
   c. watch a video of proper exercise technique.
   d. attend a training session on proper exercise techniques.
   e. do all of the above.
4. What should you do to ensure a positive learning experience?
   a. learn the basics first
   b. mentally focus during your training sessions
   c. watch for key behaviors and learning points
   d. all of the above

5. Overlearning a skill means
   a. mentally focusing while practicing.
   b. practicing until you are exhausted.
   c. practicing different training speeds.
   d. practicing the exercise beyond mastery.
6. Active practice involves
   a. learning each exercise beyond mastery.
   b. mentally focusing while training.
   c. receiving feedback while you train.
   d. increasing training time for each exercise.
7. Kinesthetic awareness is
   a. neither good nor bad in itself.
   b. feedback from movements of the body.
   c. watching another firefighter training.
   d. a learning point.
   e. monitoring your heart rate while practicing.
8. Feedback serves what purpose?
   a. allows you to set or modify your goals
   b. allows you to practice beyond fatigue
   c. keeps your motivation high
   d. conveys information about your performance
   e. a, c, and d
9. A learning point is
   a. a diagram of the fitness facility.
   b. an interview with a fit firefighter.
   c. a key behavior in successful exercise technique.
   d. focusing on a skill.
10. Feedback should be
   a. provided at least one week after your training.
   b. provided for each segment of your training sessions.
   c. can be discarded if provided by a non-firefighter.
   d. should not be provided by your coach or teammates.
   e. b and d.
11. Program planning
   a. will help you achieve your goals.
   b. is not required for experienced exercisers.
   c. is unnecessary for successful goal completion.
   d. should be done by an experienced trainer.
12. The proper time to develop a program plan is
   a. before biometric testing is done.
   b. after three months of training.
   c. after feedback is evaluated for three weeks of training.
   d. after you have set goals and learned fitness-training skills.

REFERENCES

1. Wexley, K. and Latham, G. (1981). *Developing and Training human resources in organizations* (1st ed.). (Santa Monica, CA: Goodyear).

2. Locke, E.A.; Shaw, K.N.; Saari, L. M.; and Latham, G. P. (1981). Goal setting and task performance: 1969–1980. *Psychological Bulletin*, 90, 125–152.

3. LeBoeuf, Michael. (1985). *The greatest management principle in the world*. (New York: Putnam).

4. See reference 1.

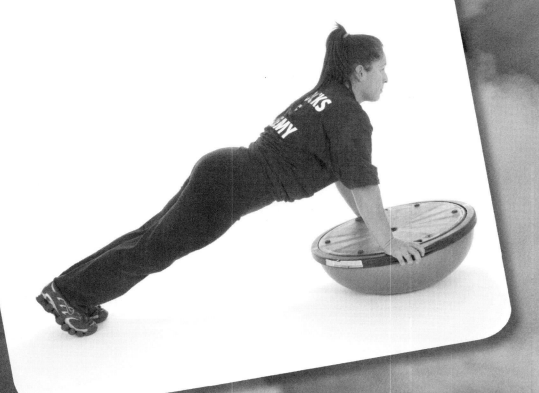

3 Learning the Skills

OBJECTIVES

Upon completion of this chapter, the firefighter will be able to

- Identify any health risk factors they have and develop workout and nutritional strategies to reduce them
- Explain the value of biometric testing in designing a training program
- List the steps involved in raising one's lactate threshold
- Understand the role that complex carbohydrates play in successful training
- List the six major nutrients and explain their role in energy production
- Describe the importance of ingesting protein and carbohydrates for the post-workout meal

- Explain the use and value of a heart rate monitor
- List the five training principles and explain their role in designing an effective training program
- Explain the role that mental training plays in maximizing performance
- Understand the concept of "centering" and explain how it is used to maximize training and prevent injury
- Determine starting points for each exercise in their program

INTRODUCTION

The creator of Famous Amos cookies was asked "Where do you start when opening a new business?" Famous Amos replied, "Start from where you are at." This chapter will cover the five components of successful fitness program design: health screening, biometric testing, fitness principles, nutrition, and mental training, **Figure 3-1**.

HEALTH SCREENING

"The health you enjoy is largely your choice."
—Abraham Lincoln

Because the primary purpose of a fitness program is to improve your quality of life and your ability to perform firefighter duties, identifying and reducing health risk factors and musculoskeletal injuries is a vital first step. Screening will identify any medical risk factors that might necessitate a referral to your physician. It will also identify any possible contra-indicated activities, enabling you to design an exercise program that includes safe activities and/or appropriate modifications.

Coronary Artery Disease (CAD)

Coronary artery disease (CAD) is caused by plaque accumulation in the heart's coronary arteries, which results in insufficient blood flow to the heart muscle. Examples of CAD disease are myocardial infarctions (heart attacks), angina (chest pain), and sudden cardiac death. Plaque accumulation in other areas of the body can result in several major health conditions. **Strokes** result from blockages of blood

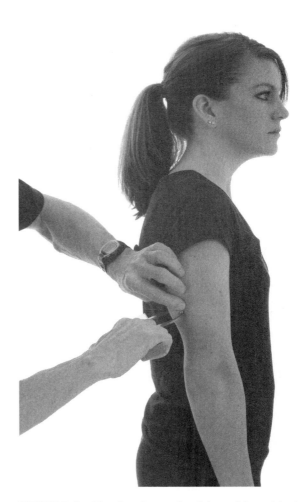

FIGURE 3-1 Feedback received from biometric testing is invaluable.

to the brain, which may result in severe brain damage and disability or death. **Peripheral vascular disease (PVD)** is a cramp-like pain in the legs resulting from blockages in blood flow to the legs. PVD can lead to gangrene and amputation of the affected extremity.

Risk Factors

Risk factors for coronary artery disease are conditions that predispose an individual to the disease. A risk factor does not guarantee that a person will develop CAD. However, when risk factors accumulate for a person the probability of developing coronary artery disease increases exponentially. The risk factors for CAD are listed below:

Risk factors that cannot be changed:

■ Heredity
■ Age
■ Gender
■ Race

Risk factors that can be changed:

■ Smoking
■ Elevated cholesterol levels
■ High blood pressure (hypertension)
■ Obesity
■ Type 2 Diabetes
■ Inactivity

The Health Screening Performance Planning Chart (see Appendix B) lists acceptable and ideal levels for all CAD risk factors.

(FFF) Only 18% of adults are free of commonly identified major risk factors, reports the Centers for Disease Control and Prevention. Heart attacks still account for 500,000 deaths per year, and 20 percent of those deaths occur in people under the age of 65.[1] More important for firefighters are the current firefighter fatality statistics related to heart attacks and stress, **Figure 3-2**.

Understanding and Reducing Risk Factors for CAD

Risk factors include both factors that can be changed and factors that cannot be changed. The risk factors that cannot be changed include the following:

1. **Heredity:** A parent or sibling who has had a heart attack before the age of 55 if a man, or 65 if a woman, predisposes an individual to CAD.

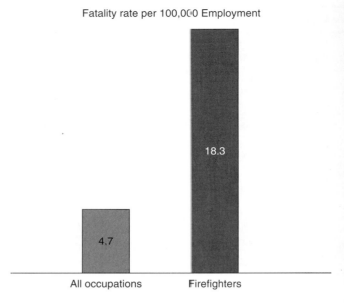

Fatality rate per 100,000 Employment

18.3

4.7

All occupations   Firefighters

FIGURE 3-2   Firefighters are about four times as likely to be fatally injured on the job compared to the average worker (U.S. Department of Labor statistics).

2. **Age:** 80 percent of fatal heart attacks and 55 percent of all heart attacks occur after the age of 65.
3. **Gender:** Men have a higher incidence of CAD than women. At about age 50, women begin to develop a similar level of risk.
4. **Race:** Because they have a higher risk for hypertension and type 2 diabetes, African Americans have an increased risk for CAD.

Risk factors that can be changed include the following:

1. **Smoking:** Overwhelming empirical evidence identifies cigarette smoking as a major positive risk factor for CAD. The risk for CAD decreases almost immediately after quitting.[2]
2. **Cholesterol:** Research has identified a strong relationship between high cholesterol levels and higher rates of CAD.[3] Cholesterol readings are broken down into three parts: total cholesterol, HDL ("good" cholesterol), and LDL ("bad") cholesterol. Each reading is important in determining CAD risk. Total cholesterol is an overall cholesterol measure. Low-density lipoprotein (LDL) cholesterol deposits plaque in arterial walls. It is often referred to as "bad" cholesterol because the more LDL in the bloodstream, the more likely plaque will be deposited along the arterial walls. LDL is strongly influenced by high levels of triglycerides, which

are a measure of fat in the blood system. Keeping total cholesterol, LDL, and triglycerides as low as possible will reduce the risk of CAD. High-density lipoprotein (HDL) removes LDL cholesterol from the blood system. The more HDL, or "good" cholesterol, you have the less LDL, or "bad" cholesterol, you will have in your blood system; therefore, a high HDL number is desirable. A *coronary risk ratio (CRR)* is computed by dividing total cholesterol by HDL cholesterol. CRR is an important measure that reflects how the body is managing individual cholesterol amounts. A low CRR is desirable.

The best approach to improving blood cholesterol levels is to reduce dietary intake of saturated fat, trans fats, and cholesterol. Diets rich in soluble and insoluble fiber (whole grains) will lower LDL, triglycerides, and total cholesterol. Increasing cardiovascular exercise also has a dramatic effect on cholesterol. Research has shown that the more calories expended doing cardiovascular exercise, the greater the effect on reducing cholesterol. There is a 2–3 percent decline in the risk of heart attack for every 1 percent reduction in total blood cholesterol.[3]

3. **High blood pressure (hypertension):** Blood pressure is the amount of arterial force or resistance the heart encounters when pumping blood to the body. *Systolic* blood pressure is the amount of pressure encountered when the heart is contracting and *diastolic* blood pressure is the amount of pressure encountered when the heart relaxes. Blood pressure is recorded as systolic over diastolic, such as 120/80. Chronic, sustained elevated blood pressure predisposes individuals to CAD by damaging the linings of the blood vessels and tissues of the heart. High blood pressure is an insidious disease. Often it has no symptoms, and most people with hypertension are not aware of it, at least initially. For each one point drop in diastolic blood pressure, a 2–3 percent drop in the risk of heart attack occurs. The easiest way to lower blood pressure is to lose weight through exercise and proper nutrition, limit sodium (salt) intake, and decrease alcohol consumption.[4]

4. **Obesity:** The percentage of Americans that are considered to be overweight or obese increased dramatically between 1960 and 2004. Johns Hopkins State University researchers state that three-quarters of the American population is expected to be overweight or obese by 2012.[5] Being overweight increases the risk for type 2 diabetes, hypertension, and high blood pressure. Weight loss has a dramatic effect on reducing blood pressure and preventing

and improving type 2 diabetes. Losing as little as five to ten pounds can make a difference by reducing the strain of excess weight on the lower back and joints. Losing weight can raise HDL levels and lower LDL and triglyceride levels. Weight control can be enhanced by resistance training, which increases resting metabolic rate.[6]

5. **Diabetes:** Diabetes is measured by the amount of *glucose* in the bloodstream (blood sugar). Prolonged and frequent elevation of glucose levels can damage the capillaries, which leads to poor circulation. Diabetes increases the risk for CAD, permanent nerve damage, kidney failure, eye problems, and high blood pressure. Type 2 diabetes rates have increased by 76 percent since 1990. Weight control, regular aerobic exercise, good nutrition, and stress reduction can improve and control diabetes.[7]

6. **Inactivity:** A sedentary lifestyle carries the same risks for CAD as smoking or high cholesterol. Twenty-two percent of Americans do not engage in any physical activity and 78 percent do not meet the minimal physical activity requirements.[7]

Reducing Risk Factors Through Exercise

Exercise and proper nutrition have the greatest effect on reducing cardiovascular risk factors. The total amount of calories expended during exercise has a direct (almost linear) effect on reducing or eliminating most health risk factors.[8]

Other Medical Conditions

If you checked any of the items in the medical conditions section of the planning chart in Appendix B, you need to obtain a physician's recommendations and release before becoming physically active or going through the biometric testing. Be sure you understand the implications of each condition and how to modify your exercise program.

Orthopedic Conditions

Even though orthopedic limitations and disease do not appear to present the same relative risk as that associated with cardiovascular function, musculoskeletal concerns are an important factor to consider when developing your exercise program. Some of these conditions require a physician's release, and you should be aware of the physiological effects and limitations that these conditions have on your

Percent of Potential Improvement in Risk Factors Achieved by Exercise

Risk Factor	Calories per week expended during exercise					
Percentage reduction in risk-factor levels	500	1,000	1,500	2,000	2,500	3,000
Triglycerides	62	83	92	96	99	100
Blood Pressure	40	61	76	83	95	99
Body Composition	23	41	57	71	88	98
HDL	16	21	35	50	76	99

exercise and firefighting performance. This text will deal with these conditions in a general sense. Contact your doctor for specific guidelines regarding each orthopedic condition you have.

Medications

The chemical reactions that occur in the body when taking medications may influence physiological responses during exercise. Various medications may alter heart rate, blood pressure, cardiac function, and exercise capacity. Your doctor should provide you with information and recommendations on the physiological effects of each medication you are on.

Family History

Awareness of one's family health history is necessary when developing a viable fitness program. The risk factors listed in the planning chart should be discussed with your physician prior to developing an exercise program.

BIOMETRIC TESTING

"Face your deficiencies and acknowledge them. But do not let them master you."

—Helen Keller

Initial biometric testing will allow you to compare your capabilities to the specific demands of a firefighting career, **Figure 3-3**. Initial testing will determine your fitness strengths and weaknesses, and enable you to determine starting points or baseline measurements for your training exercises. It will help you to set realistic and motivating training goals, allowing you to customize a training program that progresses in a safe,

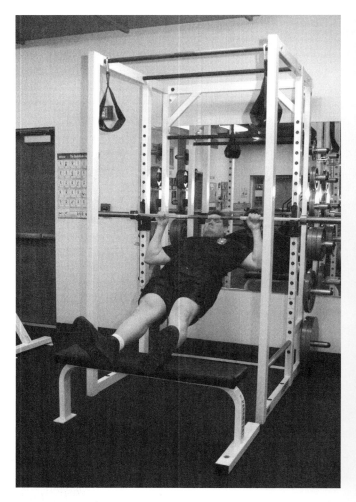

FIGURE 3-3 Initial testing provides baseline measures for your fitness program.

injury-free, productive manner Feedback provided by re-testing will help you to evaluate your goals and reset them if necessary. Re-testing will also indicate whether you are overtraining and need to scale back.

The five components of testing are

- Cardiovascular capacity
- Muscular strength and endurance
- Flexibility
- Body composition
- Functional ability

The following tests are accurate predictors of the skills and abilities required to perform the job of a firefighter. For each component, a recommended and an alternative test protocol are described. The recommended tests represent the ideal test method. The alternative tests are easy to do and do not require a lot of specialized or expensive equipment. Record the results from your tests on the biometric testing performance planning chart in Appendix A.

When performing the biometric tests, technique counts. It does you no good to perform push-ups by not going all the way down, or to perform pull-ups by going halfway down and swinging. The world is full of people touting inflated scores based on questionable testing methods. The famous anthropologist Margaret Mead said, "What people say, what people do, and what they say they do are entirely different things." Don't test for ego-inflation or to impress others; test to evaluate progress. You will gain the respect of others and of yourself.

FIREFIGHTER FITNESS FACTS

The physical ability tests described in this book are all valid measures of the requirements for firefighting. There are hundreds of tests, many of which are not valid measures of any physical ability; others are valid but are not specific for firefighting. For example, the 1.5-mile run is a common and valid test of overall aerobic fitness. However, it is not specific to firefighting. How often does a firefighter run 1.5 miles when on an emergency call? Firefighting is more of an anaerobic activity, and that is why the New York Fire Department (FDNY) stepmill protocol is used here. The 1.5-mile run is listed below as an alternative test for departments that do not have access to a stepmill or a treadmill. The fitness principle of specificity (see Fitness Principles in this chapter) states that the body responds and adapts to the type of physical demands under which it is placed. The more similar your training and testing is to the demands of a firefighting career, the more likely it is that your performance will be successful.

Cardiovascular Capacity

Cardiovascular capacity is the body's ability to meet the demands for oxygen and nutrients during physical exertion. It is measured as **VO₂ max**, which is defined as the greatest amount of oxygen that can be utilized at the cellular level. VO₂ max can be accurately measured by several submaximal or maximal tests. Submaximal tests are recommended because maximal tests require a doctor to be present.

FDNY Stepmill Protocol

Wear a heart rate monitor for this test, **Figure 3-4**.

1. The test begins with a 30-second warmup at level 3 (45 steps per minute) followed by a 3-minute exercise period at level 4 (60 steps per minute).
2. Heart rate is measured during the last 15 seconds of the test.
3. Holding on or leaning on the handrails is not allowed.
4. If at any time during the test you experience chest pain, light-headedness, or nausea, stop the test.

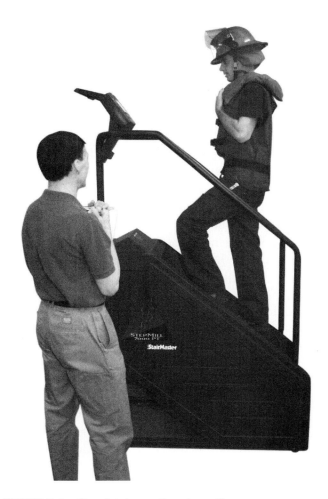

FIGURE 3-4 Candidate on the stepmill.

The following equations are used to establish VO_2 max.

Male: VO_2 max $= 1113.34 - 0.15$ (weight) $- 0.32$ (final heart rate) $- 0.54$ (age)

Female: VO_2 max $= 88.22$ $- 0.31$ (final heart rate) $- .032$ (age)

VO₂ max Classifications

Classification	VO₂ max	
	Male	**Female**
Excellent	50+	46+
Minimum level	42	38

FIREFIGHTER FITNESS FACTS

The stepmill test is one component of the biometric testing. This test is often conducted using the methods created by the New York City Fire Department (FDNY), and it is often referred to as the FDNY protocol. It is a good testing method for firefighters because it was developed and standardized using firefighters as subjects.

Alternative Test Method: Submaximal Treadmill Evaluation

1. Determine 85 percent of your predicted maximal heart rate using the following formula: 220 − age × 0.85.
2. Warm up on a treadmill at 3 mph at 0 percent grade for 3 minutes.
3. Monitor your heart rate continuously and record it during the last 15 seconds of each stage.
4. After one minute, increase the grade to 2 percent. After every odd minute increase the grade an additional 2 percent; after every even minute increase the speed by 0.5 mph. Continue until your heart rate reaches the target rate.
5. Once you have reached your target heart rate, continue the test for an additional 15 seconds to allow the heart rate to stabilize. If the heart rate does not stay at or below the target heart rate during this period then end the evaluation at the stage reached.
6. Remain on the treadmill for a cooldown for 3 minutes at 3 mph, 0 percent grade.
7. Record the time spent and refer to the VO_2 max determination listed in the table to the right.
8. Determine the VO_2 max classification.

VO₂ max Determination: Submaximal Treadmill Method

Time (minutes)	VO₂ max	Time (minutes)	VO₂ max
1:00	31.15	6:00	57
1:30	33.6	6:30	58.8
2:00	35.35	7:00	61.2
2:30	39.55	7:30	63.3
3:00	43.4	8:00	65
3:30	45.15	8:30	68.2
4:00	46.5	9:00	70.7
4:30	50	9:30	73.1
5:00	52.8	10:00	74.9
5:30	54.9		

Alternative Test Method: 1.5 Mile Run

The 1.5 mile run is a good alternative for departments that do not have access to a stepmill or treadmill. Although it is not as specific to firefighting as the previous two tests, it is an excellent measure of overall cardiovascular fitness.

1. Equipment needed is a stopwatch (or the minute hand of a watch) and a clipboard with a recording sheet and a pencil.

1.5 Mile Run Ratings

Time (minutes)	VO₂ max	Time (minutes)	VO₂ max
7:30	73.5	11:00	47.57
8:00	68.85	11:30	44.9
8:30	64.5	12:00	42.6
9:00	60.55	12:30	40.39
9:30	56.88	13:00	38.36
10:00	53.48	13:30	36.54
10:30	50.40	14:00	34.82

2. Use a quarter-mile track or measure a 1.5 mile distance with starting and finishing points.

3. Record your starting time.

4. Mark off laps if using a quarter-mile track or distance shorter than 1.5 miles.

5. Record your finishing time.

Resting Heart Rate (RHR)

An individual's **resting heart rate (RHR)** is a good indication of his or her cardiovascular fitness level. High fitness levels are associated with lower resting heart rates. The amount of blood pumped by the heart with each beat is known as **stroke volume**. As one's conditioning level increases, the heart becomes stronger and pumps more blood with each beat. Thus, a stronger heart doesn't have to beat as often as a nonconditioned heart to deliver the same amount of blood to the working muscles. The average nonconditioned adult has a RHR of 70–80 beats per minute. Highly conditioned aerobic athletes such as elite marathon runners and endurance cyclists have low RHRs (30–40 beats per minute). To determine your resting heart rate, use a heart rate monitor or manually count the beats for one minute, **Figure 3-5**. For manual determination, use your fingers to count the pulse at your wrist or at the carotid artery on the side of the neck. Resting heart rate should be measured when you first wake up, before you get out of bed in the morning. Pulse checks taken at midday or afternoon are not regarded as a true measure of resting heart rate because you have been performing **activities of daily living (ADL)** and your pulse will be elevated even when sitting. Record your resting heart rate for three days in a row and then average the readings. If your RHR is going up, it could indicate that you are overtrained

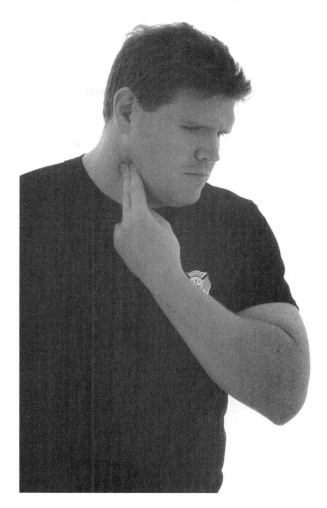

FIGURE 3-5   Manually checking heart rate.

or ill. See Chapter Five for directions on treating overtraining.

Muscular Strength and Endurance

Push-ups: Method: Upper body strength and endurance is measured by the two-minute push-up test, see **Figure 3-6** on the following page.

1. Start in the *up* position with head in a neutral position.

2. Hold the body with the back, hips, and head in alignment.

3. Do the push-up in a straight arm position and in time with the cadence of a metronome, one beat up and one beat down.

4. Set the metronome at a speed of 80, allowing for 40 push-ups per minute.

Resting Heart Rate Classifications

bpm = beats per minute

Category	RHR
Olympic-level endurance athlete	30–45 bpm
Excellent	50–54 bpm
Good	<60
Average nonconditioned adult	70–80 bpm

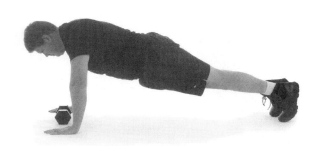

FIGURE 3-6A Push-up test—starting position.

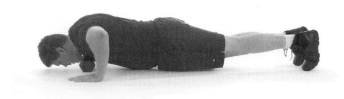

FIGURE 3-6B Push-up test—ending position.

5. Lower the torso down far enough that you could touch a 5"-high cup or a partner's fist on the floor.

6. Record the number of push-ups completed in two minutes.

7. Stop the test when you (a) reach 80 push-ups, (b) perform 3 consecutive incorrect push-ups, or (c) you cannot maintain continuous motion with the metronome.

Push-ups Minimum Standards for Firefighters		
Age (years)	Male	Female
18–35	42	20
36–52	36	15
53+	29	11

Curl-ups: The ability to transfer force generated by your lower body into the execution of firefighting duties is essential for firefighting. Your core body strength is measured by performing as many curl-ups as possible in three minutes.

1. Bend your knees at a 90-degree angle, with the hands cupped over the ears, **Figure 3-7**. The feet are secured by a bar or another individual, but the holding or bracing of the knees is not allowed.

2. Initiate the curl-up by flattening the lower back and contracting the abdominals until the trunk reaches a 45-degree angle to the floor.

3. Lower your trunk to the floor in a controlled manner until the upper back touches the floor. Rocking or bouncing is not permitted.

4. Perform the curl-ups in cadence with the metronome, one beat up and one beat down.

5. Set the metronome at a speed of 60, allowing for 30 curl-ups per minute.

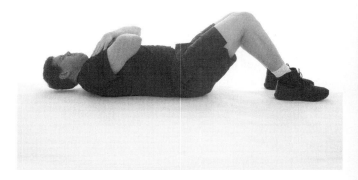

FIGURE 3-7A Curl-up test—starting position.

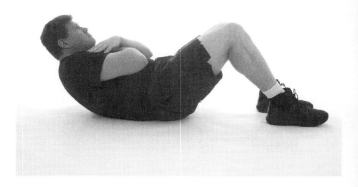

FIGURE 3-7B Curl-up test—ending position.

Curl-ups Minimum Standards for Firefighters

Age	Male	Female
18–34	70	70
35–50	50	50
51+	36	36

6. Stop the test when you (a) reach 90 curl-ups, (b) perform three consecutive incorrect curl-ups, or (c) you cannot maintain continuous motion with the metronome.

Hand-Grip Strength

The hand-grip test evaluates grip strength. A Jamar Hydraulic Hand Dynamometer is used for this test.

1. Test each hand three times by squeezing the hand-grip dynamometer in a gradual manner.

2. Hold a maximum squeeze or contraction for 2–3 seconds, then release gradually.

3. Swinging or pumping of the arm is not allowed, and the device must be held without jerking.

4. The arm must be held next to the body at a 90-degree angle. Alternate testing attempts between hands.

5. The highest of the three trials is recorded.

Bench press: The bench press is used to assess upper body strength, **Figure 3-8**. **One repetition maximum (1RM)** is the maximum amount of weight that can be lifted for one repetition. However, lifting the maximum amount of weight can lead to injury, so testing is done by using a weight that allows approximately ten repetitions.

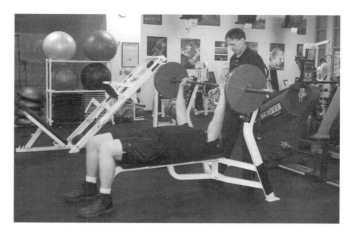

FIGURE 3-8 Bench-press test.

1. Using a spotter for safety, put enough weight on the bar that allows for performance of approximately ten repetitions (10RM).

2. Start by lying flat on the bench with your feet planted firmly on the ground.

3. Keep your back on the bench and feet firmly on the floor throughout the execution of the lift.

4. Center your grip on the bar, hands slightly wider than shoulder width. Too wide a grip will place severe stress on the shoulder joint and could lead to injury.

5. The eyes should always be open and focused on a point directly overhead.

6. Start the lift by slowly unracking the bar. If you wish, ask a partner for a lift-off and spot.

7. Slowly lower the bar to the chest, taking about 2 seconds. Generally, men should lower the bar to the nipple line, whereas women should lower the bar to slightly below that level.

8. Never bounce the bar off your chest at the bottom of the lift. Striking the chest with too great a force can result in fractures to the sternum or ribs.

Hand-Grip Strength Ratings

Age (years)	20–35		36–50		51+	
Gender	M	F	M	F	M	F
Excellent	>54	>36	>51	>36	>49	>33
Above Average	46–54	31–35	47–50	31–35	42–48	28–32
Average	40–45	28–30	43–46	28–30	39–41	25–27
Below Average	<40	<28	<43	<28	<39	<25

9. After the bar touches the chest, immediately bring it back up in a controlled movement. The bar does not go straight up, but rather at a slight angle back toward the rack.

10. Repeat for as many repetitions as possible.

11. Determine the 1RM weight.

First, key the repetitions completed into the following chart:

Number of Repetitions Completed	Percentage of 1RM Factor
5	0.87
6	0.85
7	0.83
8	0.80
9	0.77
10	0.75
11	0.70
12	0.67
15	0.65

Second, divide the weight lifted by the percentage of 1RM factor. This will give an approximate 1RM weight.

Finally, divide the 1RM by body weight to determine body weight/bench press ratio.

For example, a firefighter weighing 220 pounds bench presses 200 pounds for 9 repetitions.

Step 1: Divide 200 (weight lifted) by 0.77 (1RM factor) to equal 259.7, or 260 after rounding.

The individual's approximate 1RM would be 260 pounds.

Step 2: Divide 260 (the 1RM) by 220 (individual's body weight) to equal 1.18 (body weight/bench press ratio).

Step 3: To determine the rating, key the body weight/bench press ratio into the following chart:

Bench Press 1RM Minimum Levels		
	Weight/bench Press Ratio	
Rating	**Male**	**Female**
Excellent	>1.3	>1.0
Good	1.2	0.8–1.0
Acceptable	1.0	0.7

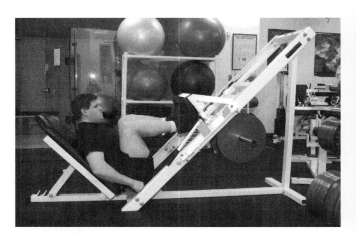

FIGURE 3-9 Leg-press test.

A male firefighter should be able to bench press his body weight at least one time and a female firefighter should be able to bench press at least 70 percent of her body weight for one repetition.

Leg press: The leg press is used to assess lower body strength, **Figure 3-9**.

1. Choose a weight that will allow ten repetitions.

2. Set the seat so that the knees are bent just over right angles.

3. Position feet about shoulder-width apart.

4. Push the platform up by pushing through the heels.

5. Extend the legs until nearly straight, avoiding locking the knees.

6. Lower the weight slowly back towards the starting position.

7. Repeat for ten total repetitions.

8. Calculate the 1RM and body weight ratio for the leg press using the same procedure that was used for the bench press.

9. Determine the rating by keying the body weight/leg press ratio into the following chart:

Body Weight to Leg Press Ratio		
Rating	**Male**	**Female**
Excellent	2.27	2.05
Above Average	1.9	1.7
Average	1.7	1.5
Below Average	>1.7	>1.5

Flexibility

Modified Sit-and-Reach Test

1. The Acuflex I tester is used and two people are needed to perform this test: one subject and one tester.

2. Shoes should be removed.

3. The subject sits on the floor with the back, hips, and head against a wall, the legs fully extended, and the bottom of the feet against the Acuflex 1.

4. The subject places one hand on top of the other (keeping the index fingers equal) then reaches forward as far as possible without letting the head, back, or hips come off the wall. The shoulders may be rounded. The technician then slides the reach indicator along the top of the box until the sliding device touches the tips of the subject's fingers, **Figure 3-10A**. The reach indicator must be held firmly in place throughout the test.

5. The subject gradually reaches forward, pushing the sliding device as far as possible along the reach indicator and holding the final position at least 2 seconds. The knees must be kept flat against the floor (**Figure 3-10B**).

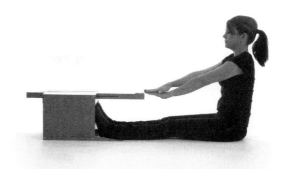

FIGURE 3-10A   Sit-and-reach test—starting position.

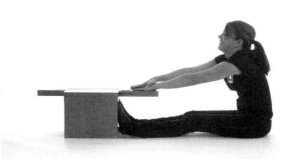

FIGURE 3-10B   Sit-and-reach test—ending position.

Modified Sit-and-Reach Test Ratings (in inches)

Men			Age Group		
Rating	**20–29**	**30–39**	**40–49**	**50–59**	**60+**
Excellent	19	17	17	17	17
Good	17	16	15.5	15.5	15.5
Above Average	16	15	14.5	14.5	14
Average	15	14	13.5	13	13
Below Average	<15	<14	<13.5	<13	<13
Women			**Age Group**		
Rating	**20–29**	**30–39**	**40–49**	**50–59**	**60+**
Excellent	20	18	17.5	17	17
Good	19	17	16.5	16	15.5
Above Average	18	16.5	15.5	15	15
Average	16	15.5	14	13	13
Below Average	<16	<15.5	<14	<13	<13

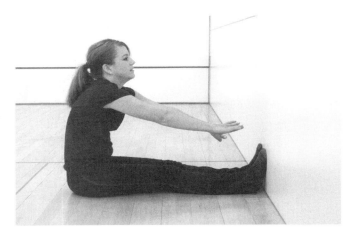

FIGURE 3-11   Sit-and-reach test—wall test.

Alternative method: The sit-and-reach wall test.

1. Remove your shoes, sit facing a wall, and keep your feet flat against the wall with your knees straight.
2. Reach forward as far as possible to touch your fingertips, knuckles, or palms to the wall and hold the position for 3 seconds, **Figure 3-11**.

Sit and Reach Wall Test Ratings	
Final reach position	Rating
Palms or better against wall	Excellent
Knuckles against wall	Above average
Fingertips touching toes	Average
Can't touch toes	Below average

Body Composition

Excess body fat has a direct effect on your performance as a firefighter. Losing excess body fat will increase your quickness and endurance, reduce the demand placed on your heart, and reduce the likelihood of injury and joint pain. Body composition is the most controversial of all the biometric tests because most methods, including underwater weighing, are at best estimates, having been validated on limited population groups. For example, bioelectrical impedance is simple to administer and interpret. However, several pretest conditions must be met such as not exercising up to four hours prior to testing, not drinking excess water, and not eating immediately preceding the test. This technique is not recommended for lean individuals because it will overestimate body fat levels, and for obese individuals because it will underestimate body fat levels.

Because measuring body composition is the most controversial of all the biometric measures, we recommend using four different methods: Dual energy X-ray scan (DEXA), skinfold calipers, body mass index (BMI), and waist-to-hip ratio. This will increase the number of feedback sources and approaches to gauging body composition. If using a DEXA scan and skinfold calipers is not feasible, a department can use BMI and waist-to-hip ratio. These two measures require only a body weight scale and a tape measure to complete.

Recommended Method 1: Dual-energy X-ray Scan (DEXA)

This is the new "gold standard" for measuring body composition. It is the ideal method because it is similar to an X-ray of the body, showing the amount and distribution of fat by location. It can be expensive; however, some companies have traveling DEXA vans that offer discounted rates for recreation centers and health clubs.

Recommended Method 2: Skinfold Measurement

This is the most common method used. To ensure accurate results, the tester must be experienced and high-quality calipers must be used, **Figure 3-12**.

Body Composition Ratings		
	Acceptable	**Ideal**
Female	<25%	<20%
Male	<20%	<15%

Recommended Method 3: Body Mass Index (BMI)

BMI uses an individual's height and weight to estimate fat levels. If a person's weight to height ratio exceeds a given number, then his or her risk for disease increases. Scientific evidence indicates that there is a significant increase in the risk for disease when BMI exceeds 25.[9] BMI is calculated by multiplying body weight in pounds by 705 and dividing this figure by the square of the height in inches. For example, the BMI for an individual who weighs 172 pounds and is 67 inches tall would be 27 (172 × 705/67^2). BMI has one major weakness: it fails to

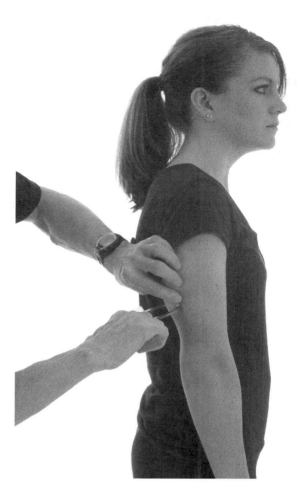

FIGURE 3-12 Skinfold test.

differentiate fat from lean body mass or note where most of the fat is located. Using BMI, athletes with a large amount of muscle mass (such as body-builders and football players) can easily fall into the moderate- or high-risk categories.

Disease Risk According to Body Mass Index (BMI)		
BMI	**Disease Risk**	**Classification**
<18	High	Severely underweight
19.9–18	Moderate	Underweight
20–24.9	Low	Acceptable
25–29.9	Moderate	Overweight
30+	High to very high	Obese

Recommended Method 4: Waist-to-Hip Ratio

This method reveals how an individual stores body fat. Scientific evidence suggests that the way people store fat affects their risk for disease. Obese individuals with a lot of abdominal fat are clearly at higher risk for many diseases, including heart disease, type 2 diabetes, and stroke.[10] Additionally, excess body weight around the midsection is a major contributor to lower back pain. The strain placed on the lower back is substantial, especially when performing firefighter tasks.

Disease Risk According to Waist-to-Hip Ratio		
Men	**Women**	**Disease Risk**
<0.95	<0.80	Low
0.96–0.99	0.81–0.84	Moderate
>1.0	>0.85	High

Functional Ability

1. Balancing: The foundation of all movement and crucial for all firefighters is the ability to balance, see **Figure 3-13** on the next page. Put on a 50-pound weighted vest and perform the following tests. Record your times for each of these tests and record them on the performance planning chart.

1. Stand on one leg for ten seconds. Then repeat on the other leg.
2. Stand on one leg for ten seconds with your eyes closed. Then repeat on the other leg.
3. On the dome side of a **BOSU** (a dome-like platform with one flat side and one rounded soft side), stand on one leg for 10 seconds, see **Figure 3-14** on the following page. Repeat on the other leg. If you do not have access to a BOSU, use an inner tube or similar object that creates an unstable surface.
4. Turn the BOSU over and stand then squat on the flat side, see **Figure 3-15** on the following page.

Ideally, you should be able to pass all four balance tests. Record your score for balance on the Performance Planning chart in Appendix B.

Alternative test: If a BOSU or Dyna Disc is not available, perform steps one and two.

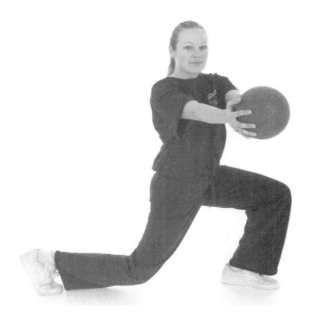

FIGURE 3-13 Lunging develops balance skills.

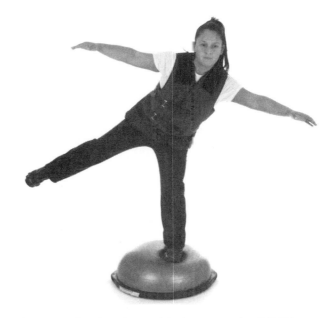

FIGURE 3-14B One-legged balance on the BOSU.

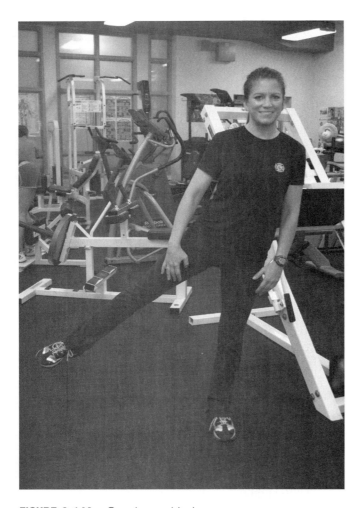

FIGURE 3-14A One-legged balance.

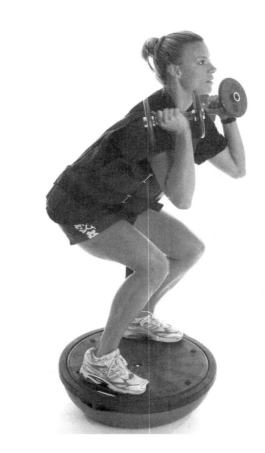

FIGURE 3-15 Squatting on the flat side of a BOSU.

2. Pull-ups: Determining maximum number of pull-ups (with palms forward) for males or chin-ups (palms toward the face) for females:

1. Elbows must be extended after each repetition is completed, and the shoulder blades must abduct (move out from the center of the body).
2. The chin must get above the bar, **Figure 3-16**. Most athletes who claim to be able to do large numbers of pull-ups actually perform half pull-ups.

Pull-up and Chin-up Ratings		
	Males (up to 225 pounds)	**Females (up to 170 pounds)**
Excellent	25+	15+
Above average	20–25	10–15
Acceptable	10–20	5–10

3. Inverted rows: The inverted row is the reverse of the bench press and primarily works the upper back and shoulder muscles involved in pulling movements.

1. lace the feet on a bench and grip a bar as if to perform a bench press. The bar should be set in a power rack at the height at which you normally bench press.
2. ith the entire body held rigid, pull the chest to the bar. The chest must touch the bar with no change in body position. Make sure there is

Inverted Row Ratings		
	Males (up to 225 pounds)	**Females (up to 170 pounds)**
Excellent	25+	15+
Good	18–25	10–15
Acceptable	10–17	4–9

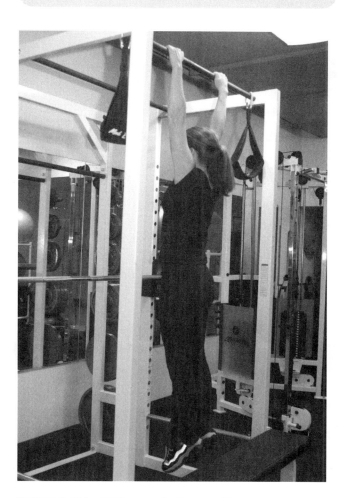

FIGURE 3-16A Pull-up—starting position.

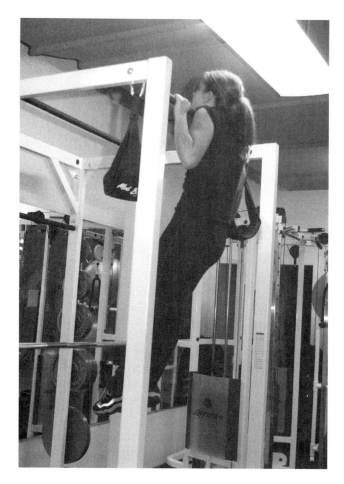

FIGURE 3-16B Pull-up—ending position.

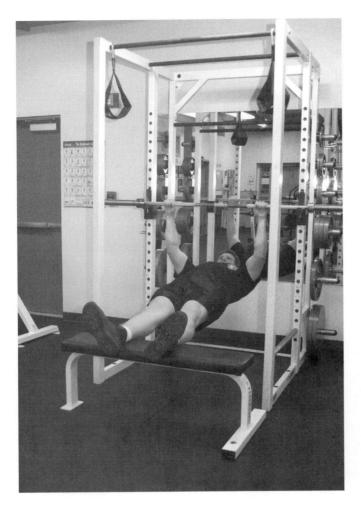

FIGURE 3-17A Inverted row—starting position.

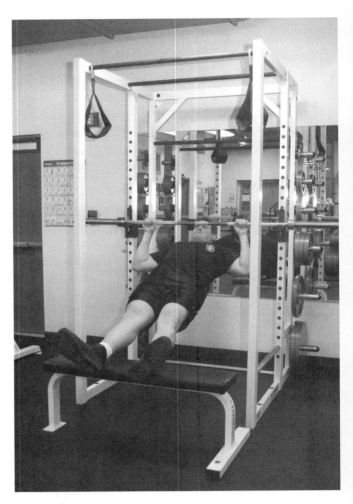

FIGURE 3-17B Inverted row—ending position.

full extension of the elbow and that the body is kept perfectly straight.

3. Count only the reps in which the chest touches the bar while the body remains straight, **Figure 3-17**.

4. Two-legged vertical jump: The Vertec brand jump tester is the recommended method. The Vertec is an adjustable device that measures standing reach height, jump height, and vertical jump, **Figure 3-18**.

1. After a five-minute warmup on a treadmill, bike, or other method, the standing reach is determined by standing directly under the measuring rods and reaching one-handed to touch the highest vane possible.

2. Jump height is determined by standing directly under the measuring rods, preloading (squatting down) then jumping without shifting the feet. The highest possible stick is touched. Swinging the arms is allowed.

3. A maximum of three trials is allowed.

5. An alternative method for this test is to estimate your vertical jump by standing next to a wall and marking your standing reach and jump height with chalk.

Vertical jump is determined by the following formula:

Vertical Jump (in inches) = jump height − standing reach

Vertical Jump Ratings

	Males (up to 225 pounds)	Females (up to 170 pounds)
Excellent	30+	20+
Good	24–30	18–20
Average	20–23	15–19

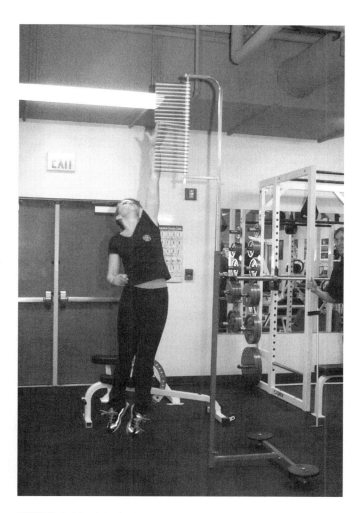

FIGURE 3-18 Vertical jump.

NUTRITIONAL CONCEPTS

"He who does not mind his belly will hardly mind anything else."

—Samuel Johnson

This section will outline the principles and guidelines of high-performance nutrition. These same principles are used by Olympic competitors, triathletes, and other athletes. It will show you what to eat and how to time your meals for maximum performance. You will have the energy to train at the high-intensity level necessary to improve your endurance and explosive power. You will be able to perform firefighter duties more efficiently and

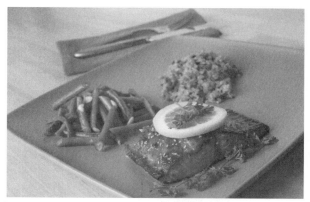

FIGURE 3-19 A diet that includes good fats, protein, vegetables, and complex carbohydrates is crucial for firefighters.

with less effort. Your risk of developing overtraining symptoms and injuries will decrease and your mental functioning will be sharp and focused, **Figure 3-19**.

Within one year's time, every cell in your body will die and a new one will replace it. These new cells are constantly developing, forming connective tissue, muscle tissue, skin, and blood. The foods you eat are the building blocks of this redevelopment process. Eating quality foods will give you the energy to train at the high-intensity level necessary to perform the job of a firefighter. Consuming poor or "junk" foods will reduce your ability to train effectively.

There are six major nutrients:

- Carbohydrates
- Proteins
- Fats
- Vitamins
- Minerals
- Water

Carbohydrates are the main energy source for the body and the most important nutrient when exercising. They are easily converted to glycogen, which the body uses for energy production. There are two types of carbohydrates: Simple carbohydrates are easily digested and quickly restore glycogen stores in the muscles. Simple carbohydrates such as potatoes, orange juice, and energy drinks and gels can supply a quick source of energy. Complex carbohydrates are slower to digest and provide energy for longer periods. Oatmeal, brown rice, and whole grains are good examples of complex carbohydrates. Among all the nutrients, they are the most powerful in affecting your energy levels, see **Figure 3-20** on the following page.

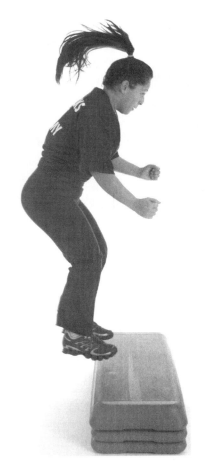

FIGURE 3-20 Complex carbohydrates will give you explosive power.

Protein is used to repair tissue damage, build the immune system, and help the body to recover from exercise. Proteins are the building blocks for all tissues, enzymes, and hormones that control our movements and metabolism. You should ingest 2 grams of protein per kilogram (2.2 lbs) of body weight per day. Good protein sources include chicken and turkey breast, egg whites, fish, lean meats, nonfat dairy products, and protein powders.

Fats carry and store fat-soluble vitamins, construct cell membranes, and play a role in the production of testosterone and estrogen. There are two types of naturally occurring fats. Saturated fats are solid at room temperature and come from animal sources. Examples of saturated fats include beef, lamb, bacon, pork, and lard products. Consuming large amounts of saturated fats contributes to many disease processes. Unsaturated fats tend to be liquid or semi-liquid at room temperature. Unsaturated fats are divided into polyunsaturated and monounsaturated. These are from plant sources and are necessary for good health and peak performance. Sources include flax seeds, avocado, walnuts, almonds, and salmon. Trans fats (partially hydrogenated fats) raise the levels of bad cholesterol (LDL) and increase the risk of heart disease.

Vitamins and minerals are not used for energy but they are needed for your body to convert macronutrients (carbohydrates, protein, and fat) to energy. Vitamins assist in the production of red blood cells, help to liberate energy from fuel stores, fight against free radicals, and help in tissue repair. Minerals help in tissue repair, play a role in maintaining a regular heart rhythm, and are necessary for muscle contraction.

Water is necessary for optimum endurance, maintaining body temperature, removing waste products, and metabolism, **Figure 3-21**. When you lose as little as 2 percent of your body weight due to dehydration your performance will decrease by 10–15 percent.

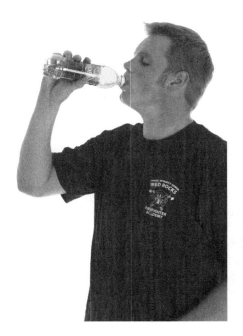

FIGURE 3-21 Water is the best drink.

High Performance Foods

Complex Carbohydrates	Proteins	Good Fats	Drinks and Seasonings
apples	beans	almonds	100% fruit juices
asparagus	brown rice and	avocado	basil
bananas	beans	canola oil	cinnamon
berries	buckwheat	fish oil capsules	green tea
black eyed peas	buffalo	flax seeds/oil	honey
broccoli	chicken breast	light tuna	orange juice
brown rice	corn and beans	natural peanut butter	oregano
brussels sprouts	corn tortillas and	olive oil	picante sauce
buckwheat	beans	peanuts	sage
cabbage	cottage cheese	salmon	salsa
carrots	egg whites	sardines	vegetable juice
cauliflower	fat-free yogurt	sunflower seeds	water
cranberries	hummus	walnuts	
dates	lentils		
kale	light tuna		
kiwi	lowfat string cheese		
mushrooms	natural peanut butter		
oatmeal	pasta and bean soup		
onions	peanuts		
oranges	salmon		
potatoes	skim milk		
quinoa	soy		
raisins	tofu		
red/green peppers	turkey breast		
spinach			
sprouted grains			
sprouts			
tomatoes			
whole-grain cereal			
whole-grain pretzels			
whole wheat			

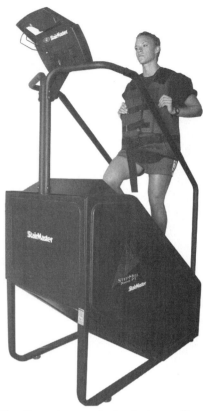

FIGURE 3-22 Complex carbohydrates will provide you with energy for high-intensity training.

Guidelines for Nutrition

1. Eat five or six meals each day. Eating every two to three hours will elevate your metabolism, keep your energy high, and promote overall body leanness.

FIREFIGHTER FITNESS FACTS

Eating five to six meals a day can be difficult for a firefighter because of the inconsistency of the daily schedule. Trying to work in a few minutes for a mini-meal between the regular meal times can be very beneficial, so it is worth the effort. Tucking a nutritional bar into a pocket or in a bag that firefighters carry can provide a method for eating a mini-meal on the go when the schedule does not permit time for preparation and sitting down to eat.

---

2. Always eat breakfast because it improves physical and mental performance. Skipping breakfast is associated with a higher risk of obesity.

3. Eat whole grain carbohydrates. Fruits, veggies, and whole grains (whole wheat bread, brown rice, and whole grain pasta) will give you more stable energy levels than processed foods like chips, soda, white bread, and candy. Sprouted grains are also good.

4. Eat fruits or vegetables with each meal. Fruits and vegetables provide you with nature's forms of antioxidants, vitamins, and minerals. Choose organic if possible.

5. Drink eight to twelve glasses of water a day. Avoid drinking a lot of fluids when eating solid food because this will slow down your digestion.

6. Always read food labels. Each gram of fat has 9 calories, each gram of protein and carbohydrate has 4 calories. Limit or avoid all foods with hydrogenated oils, saturated fat, and chemical-laden ingredients.

7. Plan ahead what you are going to eat each day. Use a cooler and some portable, reusable food storage containers for healthy snacks.

8. Keep track of your nutritional intake by keeping a food journal, **Figure 3-23**. This valuable tool will provide you with feedback on what you eat, portion size, and how much water you drink a day.

9. Proper nutrition produces high performance. Supplements are not recommended because of the side effects associated with many of them.

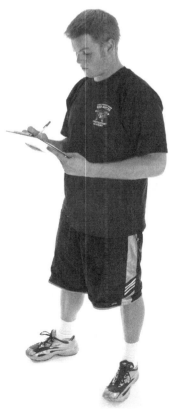

FIGURE 3-23 Tracking your nutrition with a food journal.

Pre- and post-exercise ideas for combining carbs and protein

1. Energy bar and 8 ounce sports drink
2. Two slices whole grain toast and two table-spoons peanut butter
3. One orange and half a cup lowfat cottage cheese
4. One cup cooked oatmeal with three-quarters of a cup raisins
5. One cup yogurt and quarter of a cup granola
6. Two-egg omelet with one cup fresh vegetables, one whole wheat muffin
7. String cheese and one ounce pretzels
8. Quarter of a cup nuts and a medium apple
9. Hard boiled egg and half a whole-wheat bagel
10. Whole wheat pita and half a cup canned tuna
11. Quarter of a cup soy nuts and one banana
12. Quarter of a cup sunflower seeds and one cup orange juice
13. Three ounces chicken breast and one cup cooked brown rice

10. Losing or gaining weight depends on how many calories you expend versus how many you consume. One pound of body weight equals 3,500 calories. If weight loss is desired, reduce your caloric intake by 300–500 calories per day. Do not crash diet—you will lose muscle mass and weaken yourself.

11. Strive for the 90 percent rule. Eat healthily six days per week, consuming high-performance foods. Pick one day where you eat whatever you want—nachos, pizza, cake, a piece of pie, high-caloric dinners, and so on. This will keep you from feeling deprived.

12. Eat a pre-workout meal about one and one-half hours prior to exercising. Eat complex carbohydrates and a little protein such as a whole wheat bagel with a thin layer of peanut butter on it. An empty stomach is likely to cause you to fatigue more quickly and run out of energy. Stay away from fats, as they metabolize slowly. Drink at least eight ounces of water fifteen minutes before exercise

13. During your workout, drink four to six ounces of water every ten to fifteen minutes. Drink before you feel thirsty.

14. If it is excessively hot or humid, consume more water. If your workout lasts longer than one hour use a sports drink or gel to replenish glycogen stores.

15. Consume 300–400 calories of protein and simple carbohydrates within 30 minutes after the workout. This is important because the body needs to replenish glycogen stores and start repairing tissue.

Keeping a food journal, **Figure 3-23** will enable you to track how your nutritional program is affecting your training. You will be able to modify your nutritional program if needed and gauge how many calories you consume a day. There is a sample food checklist tracking form in Appendix B.

FITNESS TRAINING PRINCIPLES

Learning and implementing sound training principles is an integral component of a successful fitness program. Training programs that include a variety of techniques have been shown to produce better results than programs that focus on a single sport or activity.[11] This section outlines an effective multidimensional approach to training that will prepare you for the demands of a firefighting career. Given demanding jobs, family, school, and life in general, most firefighters cannot afford huge blocks of time in the gym. The recommended training programs in this manual are tailored to fit the average firefighter's busy lifestyle, see **Figure 3-24** on the following page.

Fitness Training Program

The training program consists of four components:

- Cardiovascular conditioning
- Strength Training
- Functional skills
- Flexibility

Each component is described below in detail with reasons why it is important for your success as a firefighter. Use the results of your biometric testing sessions to determine the starting points for each of the training components.

Chapter Four presents several comprehensive training schedules that divide your training into four phases of increasing intensity. Included are guidelines on integrating these phases into an overall training plan that will help you achieve your fitness goals.

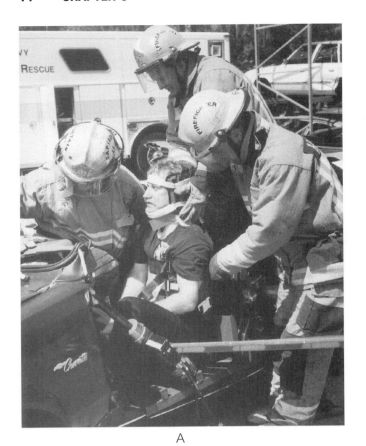

A

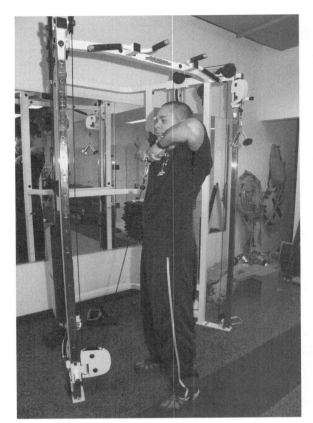

B

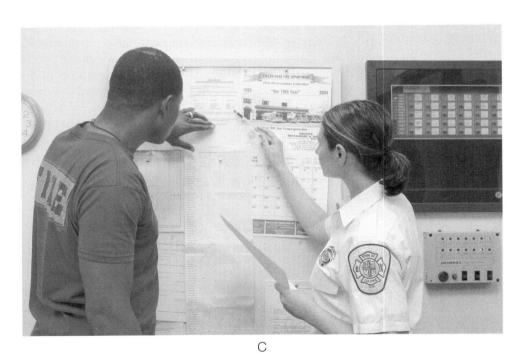

C

FIGURE 3-24 An effective fitness program can fit into the demanding career of a firefighter.

Cardiovascular Training

Cardiovascular exercise is necessary for the health, safety, and performance of all firefighters.

Firefighters should have good or excellent cardiovascular capacity. Studies have shown that the heart rate response of firefighters taken during normal firefighting tasks have been at, or near, maximum levels.[12]

The intense demands of firefighting require training both the **aerobic** and **anaerobic** energy systems. During physical activity, both systems are active at specific times depending on the intensity of the program. The aerobic system uses oxygen primarily for low-intensity training and physical activities lasting longer than three minutes. The aerobic system builds the foundation for the high-intensity anaerobic system. The anaerobic system's primary energy source is glucose that derived from carbohydrates. This system produces a high amount of energy and causes the accumulation of waste products in the muscles and blood, such as **lactic acid**. To improve your firefighting performance, it is necessary to train at levels that will increase your **lactate threshold (LT)**, that is, the point when you transition from aerobic to anaerobic energy systems. When you raise your lactate threshold, you can produce more power at a comfortable heart rate, which makes you a better performer.[13] Increasing your LT requires training at different intensity levels and gauging how your heart rate reacts at each level. To accomplish this, you need to match your heart rate with a subjective assessment of intensity.

FIREFIGHTER FITNESS FACTS

For many years we focused on finding our "target heart rate zone"—the range of heart rates optimal for improving fitness. However, there isn't one single target zone that works best for training. There are actually several zones you should spend various amounts of time training within. In addition, the formula commonly used to determine the target zone—220 minus age—can be inaccurate for any given person. Using the rate of perceived exertion scale (RPE) is your individual physiological response to exercise. RPE used in conjunction with your heart rate number is the best method.

Measuring your heart rate is best accomplished by using a heart rate monitor, **Figure 3-25**. Most cardiovascular equipment produced today has heart rate monitoring hand grips built in. However, most of these hand grips lose their accuracy as the intensity of the exercise increases because of the increased vibration. If you don't have a heart rate monitor,

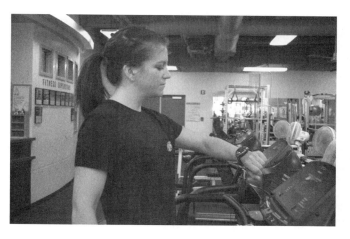

FIGURE 3-25 A heart-rate monitor will provide precision feedback for your training.

you can subjectively estimate your training zone level by using the rate of perceived exertion (RPE) method, explained below.

Cardiovascular training intensity is divided into five zones, **Table 3-1**. Determine your training or target heart rate (THR) for each of the zones by using the following procedure:

Step 1: Compute your maximal heart rate (MHR) by subtracting your age from 220.

Step 2: Determine your training heart rate range for each of the zones by multiplying your MHR by the percentage heart rate range listed. For example, a 30-year-old firefighter's heart rate for each of the zones would be the following:

Step 3: During each cardiovascular workout, compare your heart rate calculation to the **rate of perceived exertion (RPE)** or how the exercise "feels" during exercise. Note what your heart rate is and how the exercise feels.

MHR = 190	(220 − 30 = 190)
Zone 5 = 161 to 190	(190 × 0.85 = 161, 190 × 1 = 190)
Zone 4 = 142 to 160	(190 × 0.75 = 142, 190 × 0.84 = 160)
Zone 3 = 123 to 141	(190 × 0.65 = 123, 190 × 0.74 = 141)
Zone 2 = 95 to 122	(190 × 0.50 = 95, 190 × 0.64 = 122)
Zone 1 = <94	(190 × 0.49 = 94)

Table 3-1 Training Intensity Zones

Zone	Heart Rate Range	Rating of perceived exertion (RPE)
Zone 5	85–100 % of MHR	Extremely difficult. Can be sustained for very short periods.
Zone 4	75–84 % of MHR	Hard. Can be sustained from 10 to 12 minutes.
Zone 3	65–74 % of MHR	Moderate to hard. Can be sustained up to 35–40 minutes.
Zone 2	50–64 % of MHR	Moderate. Can be sustained for long periods (60 + minutes)
Zone 1	< 50 % of MHR	Easy Warm-up level.

MHR = Maximal Heart Rate (220-age)

RPE = Rate of perceived exertion or how the exercise feels.

Step 4: Recalculate your heart rate ranges.

Once you have matched your heart rate to RPE for each of the training zones, recalculate the target heart rate range for each zone if necessary. For example, if a 40-year-old firefighter's heart rate is 140 with a RPE of "moderate to hard," then both numbers of the heart rate training zone range would increase by 7 beats, changing from 117–133 to 123–140. If the firefighter's heart rate was 112 with an RPE of "moderate to hard," both numbers would drop by 5 beats to 112–128.

Cardiovascular Exercises

As your fitness levels improve, you will be able to train at higher intensities for longer periods. It is important to determine your heart rate and RPE for each training session. As your lactate threshold increases, you will be able to train at a higher heart rate level with a lower RPE.

Chapter Four introduces the concept of periodization. Detailed plans are presented on how to safely progress your workouts from low to high intensity.

Moderate intensity training (30 minutes)
Fitness level: All levels
1. Warm up for 5 minutes at zone 1
2. Minutes 6–27 go to zone 2
3. Minutes 28–30 go to zone 1

Pyramid (32 minutes)
Fitness level: Above average to excellent
1. Warm up for 5 minutes at zone 1
2. Minutes 6–10 go to zone 2
3. Minutes 11–15 go to zone 3
4. Minutes 16–18 go to zone 4
5. Minutes 19–23 go to zone 3

6. Minutes 24–30 go to zone 2
7. Minutes 31–32 cool down

Interval (20 minutes)
Fitness level: Good to excellent
1. Warm up for 3 minutes at zone 1
2. Minutes 4–5 go to zone 2
3. Minute 6 go to zone 1
4. Minutes 7–9 go to zone 3
5. Minute 10 go to zone 2
6. Minutes 11–13 go to zone 4
7. Minute 14 go to zone 2
8. Minutes 15–16 go to zone 5
9. Minutes 17–18 go to zone 3
10. Minutes 19–20 go to zone 1

Scott drills (31 minutes)
Fitness level: High

NOTE

This workout was named after the inventor, Jennifer Scott, firefighter in Cunningham Fire District

Perform the following exercises in order:
1. Treadmill at level 1 for 2 minutes
2. Stepmill climb w/weighted vest for 3 minutes
3. Stepmill backwards climb for 1 minute
4. Treadmill run/walk at 8% incline for 3 minutes
5. Versa Climber or Elliptical for 2 minutes
Repeat steps 2–5 two more times.
6. Cool down on bike for 2 minutes

Strength Training

There is no doubt that **strength training** will enhance your performance. Research has shown that athletes enjoy an increased "time to exhaustion" after following a strength-training program.[13] The main purpose of strength training for firefighting is to increase your ability to produce power, **Figure 3-26**. Appropriate strength training will also reduce injuries, decrease fatigue, and enhance your cardiovascular capacity.[13,14] Low levels of muscular strength contribute to the high incidence of muscular sprains, strains, and back injuries among firefighters. Firefighters have to be able to pull, drag, and carry heavy loads. Muscular strength is defined as the maximal amount of force a muscle or group of muscles can exert in a single contraction. Muscular endurance is defined as the ability of the muscle to perform repeated contraction for a prolonged period of time.

Strength provides the foundation on which power and endurance are built. A firefighter with high muscular strength can sustain high-intensity work longer, work more effectively, efficiently, safely, and at a lower stress level. Most firefighter injuries are associated with a lack of or insufficient muscular strength.

> **PERFORMANCE POINT**
>
> Some muscle soreness should be expected after exercise, especially if you're working at an intense level. Muscle soreness is caused by the microscopic breakdown of muscle tissue from intense exercise. The subsequent repair helps you get stronger as the muscle adapts to the increased demand.

RECOMMENDED RESISTANCE TRAINING EXERCISES FOR FIREFIGHTERS

Resistance training exercises are divided into primary and secondary exercises.

Primary exercises develop overall strength, endurance and power capability. These exercises improve all firefighter duties, including dragging and carrying victims, advancing hoselines, climbing ladders and stairs, carrying equipment, breaching ceilings and walls, and raising ladders.

Secondary exercises train muscles and skills that support the major muscle groups used in the primary upper body exercises. These muscles act as stabilizers and assistors, facilitating smooth and controlled movement for the major muscle groups.

Primary Lower Body Exercises

Squats

Muscles involved: Quadriceps, hamstrings, gluteus muscles, abdominals, lower back muscles.

Equipment and variations used: Olympic bar, power rack, fit-ball wall squats, "sissy squats," hack squats.

Related firefighter tasks: Dragging and carrying victims, climbing ladders and stairs, carrying equipment, breaching ceilings and walls, raising ladders.

Performance notes: Keeping the body in a neutral position is crucial, with chest out, eyes looking straight forward. The bar should be placed on the upper back and not on neck. Move the hips back when descending (sit on a chair). Feet placement is slightly wider than shoulder width with toes pointed out slightly. Smith machine squats place more stress on knees and ankles than free weights. Knees should not bow in or out during performance.

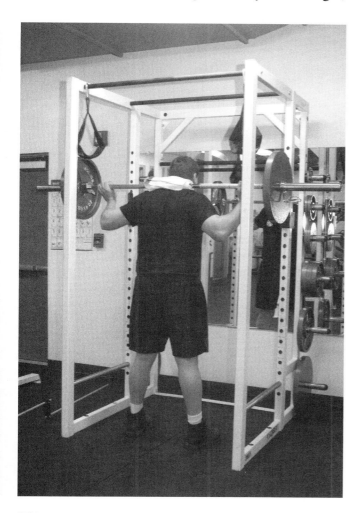

FIGURE 3-26 Multi-joint exercises like squatting develop overall body power.

Leg press

Muscles involved: Similar muscular demands as the squat but to a lesser degree. Less involvement of the abdominals and lower back. Firefighters with lower back problems might prefer this exercise to the squat.

Equipment and variations used: Leg-press machine.

Related firefighter tasks: Dragging and carrying victims, climbing ladders and stairs, carrying equipment, breaching ceilings and walls, raising ladders.

Performance notes: Feet slightly wider than shoulders on the platform, with toes pointed slightly out; hips should remain in contact with seat pad throughout the lift. High foot position emphasizes gluteus muscles, lower foot position emphasizes quadriceps. Lower foot position places more stress on knees.

Lunge

Muscles involved: Similar muscular demands as the squat with a greater emphasis on the gluteus maximus and gluteus medius. This is an excellent exercise for training balance and kinesthetic awareness (awareness of the body in motion), which are involved in all firefighting tasks.

Equipment and variations used: Barbells, dumbbells, and bodyweight.

Related firefighter tasks: Balancing in confined spaces, dragging and carrying victims, climbing ladders and stairs, carrying equipment, breaching ceilings and walls, raising ladders and advancing hoselines.

Performance notes: Body should remain in neutral position at all times; taking a big step forward when descending helps the front knee to stay over the foot. Back knee stops one inch from the floor. Motion must be controlled for both descent and ascent. Using dumbbells trains the grip and removes stress from spine.

Partial deadlifts

Muscles involved: Best overall exercise for hamstrings. High muscular involvement of the hamstrings, gluteus maximus, and gluteus medius.

Equipment and variations used: Barbells, dumbbells, wooden stick.

Related firefighter tasks: Enhances a firefighter's ability to pick up and set down objects from ground level. Trains the body to maintain neutral position for lifting and bending tasks such as victim carry and rescue and hauling heavy objects.

Performance notes: Proper performance is contingent on being in neutral position with chest out and a slight bend in the knees, hinging forward at the waist with the hips moving back when descending.

The legs remaining in static position with a slight bend in the knees.

Bench step-ups

Muscles involved: Excellent exercise for conditioning the gluteus muscles, quadriceps, and hamstrings. Balance and coordination skills are also challenged.

Related firefighter tasks: Carrying objects up stairs, stepping onto uneven surfaces, climbing steps, raising a ladder.

Equipment and variations used: Bench or step platform, dumbbells, and weight bar.

Performance notes: Movement must be controlled (especially on the return to the ground) to protect the knees and the lower spine. This exercise may be contraindicated for firefighters with back or knee problems. Proper performance is contingent upon being in neutral position with head looking straight forward and chest out.

Secondary Lower Body Exercises

Leg curl

Muscles involved: Hamstrings and gastrocnemius (outer calf muscle).

Equipment and variations used: Lying and standing leg-curl machines.

Related firefighter tasks: Breaching a ceiling and wall, raising a ladder, backing down stairs, stabilizing the body when operating a hose and nozzle.

Performance notes: The hips should remain in contact with the platform and the lower back should not hyperextend when performing this exercise. Controlled motion in both directions is important.

Seated calf raise

Muscles involved: Soleus and gastrocnemius (inner and outer calf muscles).

Equipment and variations used: Seated calf-raise machine.

Related firefighter tasks: Off-balance and uneven stance tasks, breaching a ceiling and wall, raising a ladder.

Performance notes: One-third of the foot should be on the foot bar. This allows the heel to drop for a full stretch and thus greater development. The resistance pads should be placed on the thighs and not on the knees. A full range of motion is necessary for optimal development.

Straight-leg calf raise

Muscles involved: Gastrocnemius and soleus (outer and inner calf muscles).

Equipment and variations used: Standing calf-raise machine, sliding calf-raise machine, leg press, staircase, and dumbbell.

Related firefighter tasks: Off-balance and uneven stance tasks, breaching a ceiling and wall, raising a ladder.

Performance notes: One-third of the foot should be on the foot bar of the standing calf-raise machine, leg press, or staircase. This allows the heel to drop for a full stretch and thus greater development. Neutral position must be maintained at all times. The safety catch must be in place when performing calf raises on the leg-press machine. When using a staircase, perform the exercise one leg at a time, holding a dumbbell in the hand that is on the same side as the working leg.

Knee extensions

Muscles involved: Quadriceps.

Related firefighter tasks: Breaching a ceiling and wall, raising a ladder, climbing stairs, pushing objects.

Equipment and variations used: Seated leg-extension machine.

Performance notes: This exercise should be limited to the upper half of the range of motion with the knees not locked straight at the top. This exercise might be contraindicated for a firefighter with knee problems.

Inner/outer thigh and hip movements

Muscles involved: Inner and outer thighs, gluteus maximus, and gluteus medius.

Related firefighter tasks: Stabilizing the body when in bent over and twisted positions.

Equipment and variations used: Seated or standing hip machine.

Performance notes: Body must be stabilized to avoid twisting of the back. Leg or hip should not be raised too high.

Primary Upper Body Exercises

Rowing

Muscles involved: Latissimus dorsi, trapezius, teres major, rhomboideus, infraspinatus, rear deltoids, and biceps.

Related firefighter tasks: Hose pull, ceiling breach and pull, dragging a victim, extending a ladder, clearing debris, vehicle extraction.

Equipment and variations used: Barbells, dumbbells, rowing machine.

Performance notes: Excellent exercise for the back. The dumbbell row can be performed with the knee and hand on the bench or with the hand on the bench and the feet on the floor. Barbell rows increase the risk of lower back injury because the back is not supported. Chest must be out and knees bent when rowing with a barbell. Machine row can be performed with one or two hands.

Bench press

Muscles involved: Pectorals, triceps, frontal deltoids.

Related firefighter tasks: Breaching a ceiling and wall, raising a ladder, pushing objects.

Equipment and variations used: Flat bench, barbells, dumbbells, chest-pressing machine.

Performance notes: Grip width should not exceed one and one-half times shoulder width to avoid deltoid stress. Hips should remain in contact with bench at all times.

Incline press

Muscles involved: Upper pectorals, triceps, frontal deltoids.

Related firefighter tasks: Breaching a ceiling and wall, raising a ladder, pushing objects.

Equipment and variations used: Incline bench, barbells, dumbbells, incline pressing machine.

Performance notes: Grip width should not exceed one and one-half times shoulder width to avoid deltoid stress. Bench incline should not exceed 30 degrees. Higher inclines shift emphasis to deltoid.

Deadlift

Muscles involved: Latissimus dorsi, trapezius, gluteus muscles, hamstrings, quadriceps, spinal erectors, rectus abdominis, forearm-gripping muscles, teres major, rhomboideus major.

Related firefighter tasks: Hose pulling, carrying equipment, picking up equipment, ceiling breach and pull, carrying and dragging a victim, extending a ladder, clearing debris, vehicle extrication.

Equipment and variations used: Barbells, weight plates, power rack.

Performance notes: The overall best exercise for the back. The body must be kept in neutral position throughout the lift: chest is out, lower back and abdominals tight, with knees bent. Avoid rounding the back at any time. Lift can be performed in the power rack with the bar elevated off the floor. Any shrugging of the shoulders should be done in a straight up and down motion—never "roll" the shoulders because this will damage the rotator cuff.

Shoulder press

Muscles involved: Deltoids, triceps.

Related firefighter tasks: Raising ladders, setting fans, handling hoselines, raising arms, pushing pike poles, and handling tools up a ladder.

Equipment and variations used: Vertical bench, barbells, dumbbells, shoulder-pressing machine.

Performance notes: All pressing movements should be done in front of the body because pressing behind the neck places stress on the rotator cuff.

Close-grip press

Muscles involved: Triceps, inner pectorals, frontal deltoids.

Related firefighter tasks: Breaching a ceiling and wall, raising a ladder, pulling a hose.

Equipment and variations used: Flat bench, barbells, Olympic bar.

Performance notes: Grip width should be about shoulder width. A narrow grip will stress the wrists.

Chin-ups

Muscles involved: Latissimus dorsi, trapezius, teres major, rhomboideus, infraspinatus, rear deltoids, and biceps.

Related firefighter tasks: Hose pull, ceiling breach and pull, dragging a victim, extending a ladder, clearing debris, vehicle extrication.

Equipment and variations used: Chinning bar, weight attachment belt.

Performance notes: Chin should clear the top of the bar at the top of the movement and the arms should be close to full extension at the bottom of the movement. Body should remain steady without swinging. The bar should always be pulled up to the front of the body. Pulling up to the back of the neck stresses the shoulders.

Secondary Upper Body Exercises

Pull-downs

Muscles involved: Latissimus dorsi, trapezius, teres major, rhomboideus, infraspinatus, rear deltoids, and biceps.

Related firefighter tasks: Breaching a ceiling and wall, raising a ladder, dragging a victim.

Equipment and variations used: Cable pull-down machine with various attachments.

Performance notes: The bar should always be pulled in front of the body to upper chest level. Pulling behind the neck stresses shoulders. A wide grip on the bar reduces the range of motion and is less effective. A palms-up, narrow grip allows greater involvement of the biceps.

Seated row

Muscles involved: Latissimus dorsi, trapezius, teres major, rhomboideus, infraspinatus, rear deltoids, and biceps.

Related firefighter tasks: Breaching a ceiling and wall, raising a ladder, pulling a hose, grip strength for victim drag.

Equipment and variations used: Cable seated row machine.

Performance notes: The body should be kept at a 90 degree angle (the back is never rounded) when rowing. The pull is always in front of the body to upper chest level. A wide grip is less effective. Supinated grip (palms up) allows greater involvement of the biceps. A wider bar allows greater contraction of the back muscles. A high elbow position emphasizes the upper back muscles.

Bicep curls

Muscles involved: Bicep, forearm flexors.

Related firefighter tasks: Breaching a ceiling & wall, raising a ladder, dragging a victim.

Equipment and variations used: Dumbbells, barbell.

Performance notes: Start by holding the dumbbells at arms length with the palms facing each other. As you curl the dumbbells upward, turn the palms so they face upward. This will activate both of the bicep muscles. If you keep the palms facing up during the exercise, only one of the bicep muscles will be activated. When lowering the dumbbells, reverse this process so the palms face each other upon completion of the exercise. It is also important to keep the elbows against your sides during the exercise. This will focus the work on the bicep muscles and not on the shoulders and back muscles.

Push-downs

Muscles involved: Triceps.

Related firefighter tasks: Breaching a ceiling and wall, raising a ladder.

Equipment and variations used: Cable push-down machine.

Performance notes: Can be done overhead for variation.

Dumbbell lateral raises

Muscles involved: Deltoids.

Related firefighter tasks: Raising ladders, setting fans, handling hoselines, raising arms, pushing pike poles, and handling tools up a ladder.

Equipment and variations used: Dumbbells.

Performance notes: Dumbbells should be raised to shoulder height only. A light weight should be used and the movement controlled both directions.

Alternative Exercises

Body weight exercises are a great alternative if conventional barbells and dumbbells are not available, **Figure 3-27**. Appendix A depicts seventeen exercises that use an individual's bodyweight in combination with a weighted vest or firefighter gear for added resistance. Using the building exterior and surrounding area is another option. The Candidates Physical Abilities Test (CPAT) preparation course at Red Rocks Community College utilizes the outside stairways, hills, passageways, and ledges for a variety of firefighter-specific exercises. Every exercise has alternatives.

Functional Training

Functional training develops firefighter skills that are not trained in the other three components, see **Figure 3-28** on the following page. It is a system of specialized exercises designed to reduce injuries and develop a higher level of preparation for the job of a firefighter.

Functional training can be divided into general functional training and specific functional training. **General functional training** focuses on training the core (lower back and abdominals) and developing balance. Core training enhances all of the other components because the forces applied by your arms and legs must pass through the core of your body. If the core body is weak, much of the force is dissipated and this will result in poor performance. Balance training involves instability so that the firefighter must react to regain stability.

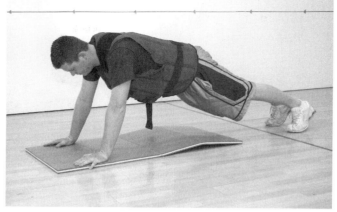

A

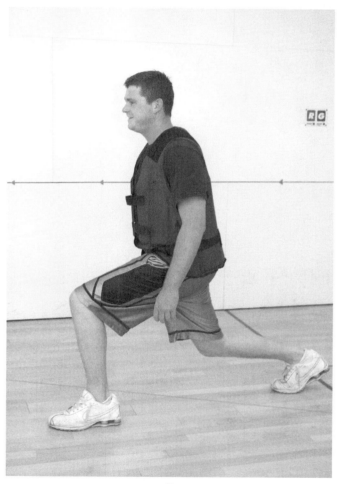

B

FIGURE 3-27 Body weight exercises are a great option if you do not have conventional equipment.

Specific functional training focuses on training for specific firefighting tasks such as pulling a hose, dragging a mannequin, breaching a ceiling, and so on.

You can use the bench press to develop general upper-body strength, but if you cannot perform body-weight exercises such as push-ups, chin-ups,

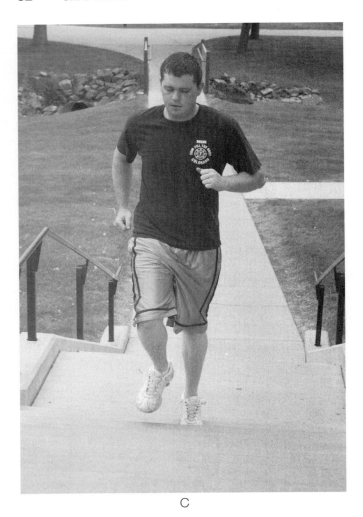

C

FIGURE 3-27   Continued.

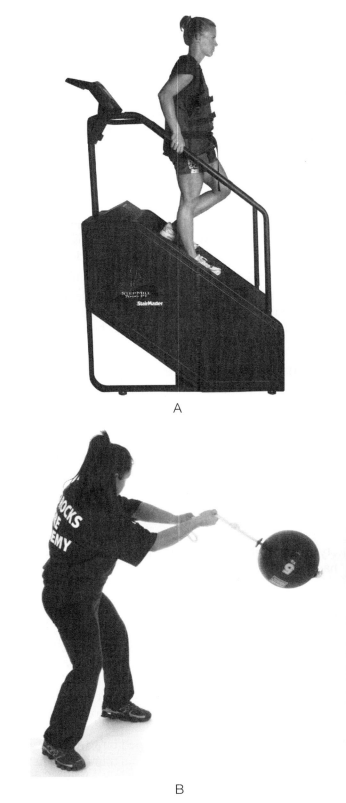

A

B

FIGURE 3-28   Functional training develops firefighting skills.

and dips, then you are not functionally strong and more likely to be injured. A good functional strength program employs tried and true strength exercises such as the bench press and front squat and then transforms the strength developed into functional strength through movements such as stability ball push-ups and one-leg squats. The ability to display strength in conditions of instability is actually the highest expression of strength. Proponents of machine-based training systems argue that machine-based training is safer. However, most weight training machines are not defined as functional because the load is stabilized for the lifter by the machine. This lack of **proprioceptive** input (internal sensory feedback about position and movement) in machine training does not prepare firefighters for actual firefighting situations.

The CPAT and the Firefighter Challenge are tests of functional capacity. They require the firefighter or candidate to apply the strength and conditioning they have developed in order to accomplish several tasks that are specific to firefighting.

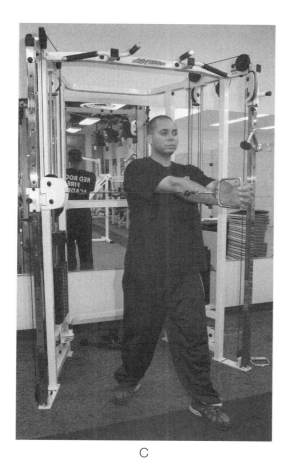

C

FIGURE 3-28 Continued.

General Functional Training Exercises

Crunches

Muscles involved: Rectus abdominis (front part of abdominal area).

Equipment and variations used: Flat surface, Fit Ball, medicine ball. Advanced version: Fit ball crunch with medicine ball, Russian twist on Fit Ball using a medicine ball.

Performance notes: Shoulders should be lifted approximately three to four inches off the ground. Performing crunches on a Fit Ball enables one to achieve a greater stretch at the bottom position. Holding a medicine ball at chest level increases the difficulty level.

Hyperextensions

Muscles involved: Gluteus muscles, hamstrings, spinal erectors.

Equipment and variations used: Flat surface, Fit Ball, medicine ball BOSU superman (laying face down with arms and legs off floor).

Performance notes: Shoulders should be lifted approximately three to four inches off the floor. Full range of motion should be used when performing with a Fit Ball.

Holding a medicine ball at chest level increases the difficulty level.

SPECIFIC FUNCTIONAL EXERCISES FOR FIREFIGHTING

Listed below are several specific functional exercises for firefighting.

If your department does not have the ideal equipment listed, think about the specific movements and demands of the firefighter tasks you wish to duplicate. There is always an alternative.

Firefighting Task	Ideal Exercise	Alternative Exercise
Stair climbing	Stepmill w/weighted vest	Staircase or Reebok step
Hose drag	Hose drag	Tire rope drag
Carrying saws	Carrying saws	Carrying dumbbell or paint can
Ladder raise/extn	Ladder raise/extn	Pole raise, cable pull-down
Breaching a wall	Hammer swing	Ball and rope swing, cable swing
Rescuing a victim	Dragging a mannequin	Sack or duffel bag drag
Breaching a ceiling	Pike pole raises and pulls	Knapsack level raises and pulls

Russian twist

Muscles involved: External oblique, rectus abdominis.

Equipment and variations used: Fit Ball, medicine ball.

Performance notes: This exercise should be performed face up on a Fit Ball with the torso turned completely to the side when rotating.

Incline leg raises

Muscles involved: Transverse abdominis, rectus abdominis.

Equipment and variations used: Incline abdominal bench.

Performance notes: The hips are raised three to four inches off the bench. Feet should go straight up and not back toward the head. Knees should be slightly bent.

Hanging knee raises

Muscles involved: Transverse abdominis, rectus abdominis.

Equipment and variations used: Chin-up bar.

Performance notes: The range of motion should be limited by keeping the knees flexed at a 90-degree angle. The upper body is kept as stationary as possible and the knees pulled into the chest.

Plank

Muscles involved: Transverse abdominis, Rectus abdominis, obliques, deltoids, lower back, glutes.

Equipment and variations used: Floor, Fit Ball, medicine ball, BOSU.

Performance notes: Keep the body as stationary as possible. Perform the exercise in sets, increasing the duration with each repetition.

Push-up

Muscles involved: Transverse abdominis, Rectus abdominis, obliques, deltoids, lower back, glutes.

Equipment and variations used: Floor, Fit Ball, medicine ball, BOSU fit ball push-up, medicine ball push-up, fit ball/medicine ball pushup.

Performance notes: Keep the body as stationary as possible. Perform the exercise in sets, increasing the duration with each repetition.

Balance

Muscles involved: Transverse abdominis, rectus abdominis, obliques, lower back, gluteus muscles, vestibular system, somatosensory system.

Equipment and variations used: Floor, BOSU Dyna Disc, wobble board BOSU standing and squatting, one-leg balance, Dyna disc one-leg balance, Dyna disc balance and reach.

Performance notes: The body is kept as stationary as possible. The exercise is performed in stages, starting with standing on both feet, then on one foot, then with the eyes closed. Try to increase the time spent at each stage.

Flexibility

Flexibility is defined as the capacity to move freely in every intended direction, **Figure 3-29**. Ideally, an individual should have enough elasticity to allow for full range of motion yet not so much that the joints are unstable. Stretching increases physical efficiency because a flexible joint requires less energy to move through its range of motion. When movement is compromised by tight muscle groups, performance diminishes and the risk of injury increases. A consistent and effective program of stretching can prevent and reduce the risks of injury and low back pain.

A lack of flexibility will inhibit smooth performance and increase the risk for injury for firefighters. The International Association of Firefighters (IAFF) Death and Injury Survey states that strains, sprains, and back injuries are the leading injuries for firefighters. All of these are directly impacted by a lack of flexibility.

Muscles must be warmed up prior to stretching them. Pre-workout stretching of cold muscles can reduce workout strength and performance. It also increases the risk of injury because the muscles are less pliable in a cold state. At the end of each workout, cool down by using **static stretching** to adequately recover and reduce later muscle soreness. Static stretching involves going into a stretch position and holding it at your point of limitation for 15–30 seconds. Avoid bouncing as this will tighten muscles.

Flexibility exercises

(illustrations of the following stretches can be found in most exercise science textbooks or the American

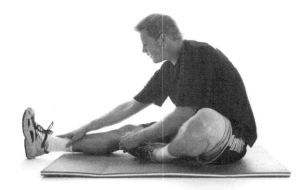

FIGURE 3-29 Flexibility is an important part of a fitness program.

Council on Exercise Personal Trainer Manual, Third Edition)

Duration: hold each stretch 20–30 seconds

Repetitions: Perform each stretch one time2

Lower Body Stretches:

Seated hamstring stretch: Standing calf stretch, straight leg

Seated inner thigh stretch: Standing calf stretch, bent leg

Lying hip stretch: Hip flexor stretch

Standing quadriceps stretch: Groin straddle

Lying lower back: Lying spinal twist

Upper body stretches:

Shoulders: cross arm in front of chest

Triceps: behind neck stretch

Shoulders: straight arms behind back

PERFORMANCE POINT

For a long time it was recommended that individuals should stretch before a competition or before their workouts. It was thought that stretching reduces the incidence of injury and pulled muscles. This recommendation was given mostly out of intuition and was not based on any hard data. Now it is thought that warming up by increasing blood flow to muscles is a better way to prepare for exercise and prevent injury. According to experts, warming up increases blood flow, speeds up nerve impulses, and assists in the removal of waste products. All stretching should be done at the end of each workout.

Training Principles

1. **Specificity:** The body responds and adapts to the type of physical demands under which it is placed. The more similar your training is to the demands of a firefighting career, the more likely it is that your firefighting performance will be successful.[12]

2. **Overload:** The body will adapt to an increase in physical demands placed on it. For continued improvement you have to gradually make the program harder with intermittent periods of rest and recovery built in. This will allow you to avoid overtraining and injury, yet provide enough challenge to allow adaptation to occur.

3. **Reversibility:** The body's fitness level will decline if you discontinue your exercise program. Without appropriate exercise, muscles become smaller and weaker, the cardiovascular system becomes less efficient, and flexibility levels will decrease.

4. **Individuality:** The capacity of each individual to handle a given workload is unique. If you and a friend do exactly the same training in precisely the same way, you probably will not get the same results. Some individuals are "fast responders" while others are "slow responders." This is probably genetic. Women generally need more recovery time than men and older individuals require longer recovery time than younger individuals.

5. **Warm-up and Cool Down:** Always warm-up for five to ten minutes prior to beginning an exercise session. Use light running, treadmill walking, biking, and so on. A thorough warm-up will increase blood flow to joints and muscles, increasing freedom of movement and reducing the risk of injury. Cool down after the workout by stretching for five minutes and using relaxed breathing. This is the ideal way to return your body to normal after exercise.

6. **Determine your starting points:** Use the biometric testing results to determine your starting points for each of the components. This will also allow you to gauge your progress and make periodic adjustments if necessary.

7. **Balance your training:** Develop a comprehensive program that includes cardiovascular, resistance training and flexibility exercises. If you are combining strength training with other components, perform the strength training first. This will allow you to maximize strength benefits. Your starting weights are determined by your biometric testing results.

   Keep the number of strength training exercises low and focus on major muscle groups. This will ensure maximum strength for the "power" movements, which more closely simulate the actions performed in firefighting.

8. **Cycle your training:** Plan your training to include varying periods of low, high, and medium intensity levels. Rest weeks should also be planned out. This will help prevent overtraining and injuries.

9. **Keep records:** Keeping records is the best form of feedback on your training program. You will be able to determine the effectiveness of your training as well as set and modify your goals. It is amazing how many people do not keep records of their training.

10. **Train with a purpose:** One of the goals of training is to make your exercise time effective and efficient. For too many people, the gym or fitness center is a social experience with an exercise set done every fifteen minutes between sessions of conversation. Yes, there is a social

aspect to training but it should not be the focus of visiting the gym. Your focus should be on training and not on socializing. If your resistance training exercises from start to finish are taking longer than one hour to complete, you are not training hard enough or are taking too much time between exercises. The idea is to get in and out of the gym effectively and efficiently.

11. **Focus on quality training:** Many individuals train in a sloppy, inefficient manner. They cheat on the lifting and neglect the lowering. In the process they arch their backs, move their elbows, dip their shoulders, bounce the bar off their chests, and do dozens of little things that make the exercises easier. On the contrary, they should be doing little things to make the exercise harder. Harder exercises, not easier, are what stimulate muscular growth. Think progression, adding more weight when the resistance seems easier. Never sacrifice proper execution for more weight. Try to make the exercise more difficult by slowing down and eliminating as much momentum as possible. Harder exercises, not easier, are what stimulate muscle growth.

MENTAL TRAINING FOR FITNESS

"Mental toughness is essential to success."
—Vince Lombardi

Preparation for your exercise sessions and firefighting duties is much like preparation for sporting games. You mentally compare how your capabilities "stack up" with the challenge that awaits you. Similar to physical skills, mental skills need to be learned, trained, and mastered. Most great athletes acknowledge that training the mind as well as the body is necessary to achieve success.

Final results are determined by how you use mental training techniques to apply your skills. Your mind "guides" your body when exercising. It allows your body to apply the skills you have developed. Mental and muscle memory interact, and you can train them together to maximize your performance. When you strengthen your mental skills, your confidence is strengthened and your commitment is enhanced.

> **FIREFIGHTER FITNESS FACTS**
>
> Mental preparation and training is nothing new to firefighters. The firefighting profession demands that firefighters mentally prepare for every incident before arrival. Firefighters can approach fitness initiatives with this same type of "mental prep."

Principles of Mental Training

Visualization: Visualization trains you to mentally experience each event as if you were living it. Perform daily sessions in which you visualize yourself completing training sessions with perfection. By imagining yourself successfully completing each exercise, your subconscious mind will "tell" your conscious mind to perform in that manner.

When practicing, picture yourself doing the skills, then actually perform each skill, letting it unfold naturally and trusting your body to do what it has been trained to do. When you actually train or take the firefighter challenge test after first visualizing them, it will be a finalization of something you have done before.

Focusing: Focusing allows you to maximize your performance by excluding all irrelevant thoughts and emotions. A positive focus connects you totally with your performance, **Figure 3-30**. Determine what focus will work for you and use it to direct your mind when training or performing firefighter duties.

Staying focused throughout your entire training session is a challenge. You will also need to develop a refocusing strategy to respond swiftly to lapses in focus. Use the refocusing strategy to shift your attention away from worry and on to performing the next exercise.

Self-talk: Do the things you say to yourself make you feel like a failure, or do they make you feel

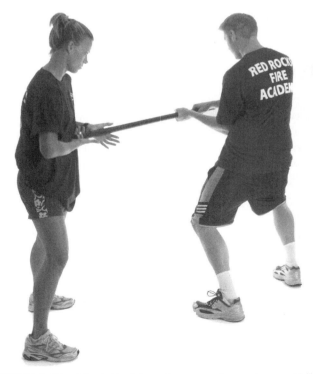

FIGURE 3-30 Mental training allows you to apply your skills.

confident and strong? All positive thoughts are constructive. All negative thoughts are destructive. The constructive force of positive self-talk will lead you to success in training and performing firefighting tasks. Examples of positive self-talk are *mantras*, phrases such as "quick feet" or "strong body" that you repeat to yourself. You can use positive self-talk as your focus points also. A good example is using the *mantra* "strong legs" when climbing stairs. Remember, only you can determine what focus points and self-talk will work for you.

Relaxation: Stress makes your mind hurry and your muscles tense up. When you are feeling stressed, slow everything down. Use breathing techniques to relax, and consciously loosen tight muscle groups. Control tension in specific muscles by tensing and then relaxing a muscle group. Repeat this process throughout the entire body. If you tense up when performing physical training or physically demanding activities, breathe deeply three or four times and focus on a positive thought. The ability to relax and maintain proper form results in less energy lost, increased confidence, and faster times, **Figure 3-31**.

Self-control: Are you willing to accept the input and advice of your coach or instructor, other candidates, or your significant other? Worry diminishes performance. Do you avoid wasting energy worrying about things beyond your control? Are you disciplined enough to use refocusing techniques to regain lost focus when necessary? Do you use relaxation techniques to calm yourself in stressful situations? Do you follow a healthy exercise and nutrition program? All of these are examples of self-control.

Centering: Centering is the breathing and focusing process that you go through to position yourself for optimal performance. Being centered allows you to transfer all of your power into your movements. Your center of mass is a spot located just below and behind your navel. When you are centered, your knees are slightly bent and your weight is evenly distributed between your feet, **Figure 3-32**. If a boxer raises his center of mass by locking his knees before throwing a punch, he cannot get his

weight or power behind the punch. If the boxer begins with a low center of mass (knees bent) and then transfers his weight by raising the center of mass as he jabs, he has the full weight of his body behind the punch. Shifting your center of mass through your body gives power to movements.

PERFORMANCE POINT

No matter how much an individual has prepared for emergency situations, the possibility of "choking" or making mistakes is a reality. Following the training plans presented in this manual will reduce this likelihood and help you to recover from mistakes. The difference between success and failure is preparation—both physical and mental.

Guidelines for Mental Training

1. Set goals for mental training as you would for physical training. The attainment of goals will increase your self-confidence and open the door to optimal performance.

2. When exercising, use strong, positive focus points. This will help you avoid distractions. Recall your best past performances and the feelings and focus associated with them. Find out what works for you. Focus on what you should be doing. Do not focus on what you shouldn't be doing.

3. Develop a refocusing strategy. When you get distracted, use simple reminders, images, or mantras to regain your focus. Refocus with positive self-talk such as "strong core" or "strong legs."

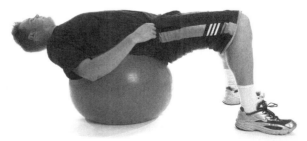

FIGURE 3-31 The cool-down after exercise is an effective time to use relaxation principles.

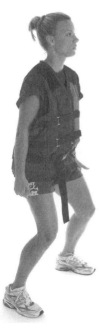

FIGURE 3-32 Proper centering position.

CASE STUDIES

Firefighter candidates Art and Jennifer set the following nutritional goals:

Goal 1: Develop a nutritional plan.

Objective: Determine total daily caloric needs.
Objective: Break down daily calories into carbohydrate, protein, and fat percentages.

Goal 2: Develop a feedback mechanism for the nutritional program.

Objective: Utilize the nutrition log in Appendix B to track their progress.

Jennifer: Body weight (bw) = 130 lbs.

Training	Calorie Calculation:	Daily Calories Needed from:		
Phase	Daily calories needed	Carbs	Protein	Fat
One	20 × bw = 2,600	65% = 1,690	15% = 390	20% = 520
Two	20 × bw = 2,600	65% = 1,690	20% = 520	15% = 390
Three	21 × bw = 2,730	65% = 1,775	20% = 546	15% = 409
Four	21 × bw = 2,730	65% = 1,775	20% = 546	15% = 409

Art: Body Weight (bw) = 200 lbs.

Training	Calorie Calculation:	Daily Calories Needed from:		
Phase	Daily calories needed	Carbs	Protein	Fat
One	20 × bw = 4,000	65% = 2,600	15% = 600	20% = 800
Two	20 × bw = 4,000	65% = 2,600	20% = 800	15% = 600
Three	21 × bw = 4,200	65% = 2,730	20% = 840	15% = 630
Four	21 × bw = 4,200	65% = 2,730	20% = 840	15% = 630

4. Make self-talk simple and positive. Remind yourself of your best performances and training sessions and your ability to perform well.

5. Prior to each exercise, visualize yourself performing with flawless technique. Analyze your performance and pinpoint any flaws. Then visualize yourself overcoming those flaws.

6. Use relaxation techniques and positive self-talk to shift your focus away from worry.

7. Your relaxation responses must be well-learned. Start by practicing firefighter skills under low-stress conditions, then under medium-stress conditons, and finally under high-stress conditions.

8. Use breathing and focusing techniques to center your body before each exercise. As you train, learn to shift your center of mass, transferring your energy into your movements.

9. Use self-talk and visualization during your days off. This will train your subconscious mind and will transfer to your actual performance.

10. Develop a support system. Your family, friends, coach, significant other, and so on will help you push through hard workouts.

11. Self-control helps you develop the mental skills required to perform your best. These skills are developed long before test day through

preparation and experiences that teach you to maintain or regain control over your mental state.

PERFORMANCE POINT

Learning to center yourself and then transferring the center of mass through your body and into the skills you are practicing or executing is the key to performing well. This skill is developed by using relaxed breathing and focus points. At first, this process will be conscious and mechanical. Thought processes often interfere with your ability to feel centered. With quality practice, the process will become quicker and automatic and you will be able to maintain freedom from distractions for longer periods. The following are

examples of positive self-talk, or *mantras*, for centering:

Loose	Controlled	Relaxed	Confident
Solid	Powerful	Balanced	Fluid
Calm	Light	Tranquil	Energetic
Peaceful	Effortless	Easy	Commanding
Clear	Smooth	Focused	Strong

Find words that are the most powerfully associated with performing at your best. Which words seem to have the strongest emotional impact on you? Those words will act as triggers to help you establish a feeling of being centered.

CHAPTER SUMMARY

A successful fitness training program is composed of health screening, initial and ongoing biometric testing, well-conceived training principles, effective mental training abilities, and a solid nutritional plan.

Initial biometric testing will determine starting points and goals for all training components. Retesting will provide feedback on program effectiveness and enable individuals to evaluate and reset goals if necessary.

Nutritional planning is necessary to meet the intense training and occupational demands of firefighting. Each firefighter's nutritional plan should be designed to meet the changes in program intensity, prevent overtraining, and reduce the occurrence of injuries. Proper meal timing, meal frequency, and water intake will increase energy and aid recovery. Maintaining a food journal will enable firefighters to track the effectiveness of their nutritional program.

The recommended firefighter fitness training program consists of four components: cardiovascular conditioning, strength training, functional skills, and flexibility/stretching. These components will develop the general conditioning and specific skills necessary for firefighters. Mental training is an integral part of every firefighter's training. A well-developed mental training program will allow the body to apply the skills developed during exercise sessions. This will strengthen a firefighter's confidence and commitment. The most crucial mental skill, focusing, is used to eliminate outside influences and concentrate on the exercise being performed. All of the mental skills are used to perfect the ability to center, which allows the transfer of lower body force into the production of power.

KEY TERMS

Activities of daily living (ADL) are everyday duties that most people perform such as walking, dressing, bathing, and so on.

Aerobic energy system uses oxygen primarily for low-intensity training and physical activities lasting longer than three minutes.

Anaerobic energy system uses as its primary energy source glucose derived from carbohydrates. This system produces a high amount of energy for short-term, high-intensity activities.

Body Mass Index (BMI) incorporates height and weight to estimate an individual's risk of cardiovascular and other major diseases.

BOSU is a dome-like platform with one flat side and one rounded soft side.

Cardiovascular conditioning utilizes exercises involving the large muscles of the body to train the heart and lungs.

Centering is the breathing and focusing process that enables one to physically position oneself for optimal performance.

Coronary artery disease (CAD) is caused by plaque accumulation in the heart's coronary arteries, which results in insufficient blood flow to the heart muscle.

Coronary Risk Ratio (CRR) is computed by dividing total cholesterol by HDL cholesterol.

Flexibility is the capacity to move freely in every intended direction.

Focusing is concentrating on a specific task by excluding all irrelevant thoughts and emotions.

Functional training develops firefighter skills not trained in other training modalities.

General functional training focuses on training the core (lower back and abdominals), balance, and reaction time.

Mantra is a short phrase or word used to help an individual focus on improving performance.

One repetition maximum (1RM) is the maximum amount of weight that can be lifted for one repetition.

Peripheral vascular disease (PVD) is a cramp-like pain in the legs resulting from blockages in blood flow to the legs.

Primary exercises develop overall strength, endurance, and power capability.

Proprioception is the ability to control and direct the body's movements when balancing and moving through space based on internal feedback.

Rating of perceived exertion (RPE) is a subjective assessment of exercise intensity.

Relaxation is using breathing techniques to relax tight muscles and dissipate stress.

Resting Heart Rate (RHR) is heart rate that is taken in a rested state. An individual's resting heart rate is a good indication of his or her cardiovascular fitness level.

Risk factors are conditions that predispose an individual to disease.

Secondary exercises train muscles and skills that support the major muscle groups used in the primary upper body exercises.

Self-control is the willingness to accept the input and advice of competent others and control one's focus to achieve a desired result.

Self-talk is words or short phrases that an individual repeats to improve performance. Examples of positive self-talk are *mantras* such as "quick feet" or "strong body."

Specific functional training focuses on training specific tasks such as pulling a hose, dragging a mannequin, breaching a ceiling, and so on.

Strength training utilizes body weight, elastic tubing, machines, barbells and dumbells to increase and maintain muscular strength and size.

Stroke is the result of blockages of blood to the brain, which may result in severe brain damage and disability or death.

Stroke volume is the amount of blood pumped by the heart with each beat.

Static stretching is holding a stretch at a set point instead of bouncing or moving.

Trans fats are partially hydrogenated fats that raise the levels of LDL cholesterol.

Visualization is mentally experiencing each exercise before performing it.

VO$_2$ max is the greatest amount of oxygen that can be utilized at the cellular level.

CHECK YOUR LEARNING

1. Centering involves
   a. focusing on the center of your body.
   b. eliminating outside distractions when you are training.
   c. transferring the force generated from your lower body into your performance.
   d. calming your emotions.
2. Strengthening your mental skills will result in
   a. your mistakes being minimized.
   b. your strength increasing.
   c. your confidence increasing.
   d. your commitment being enhanced.
   e. a, c, and d.

3. Visualization involves
   a. checking-out the training facility or test site ahead of time.
   b. seeing yourself executing your movements with perfect form.
   c. watching other people before attempting an exercise.
   d. watching successful firefighter candidates take a physical abilities test.
   e. a and b.
4. The most effective way to increase your explosive power is to
   a. raise your lactate threshold.
   b. master your ability to center yourself.

   c. develop a focus point for training.

   d. run between exercises.

5. The overload principle states that

   a. skills must be maintained or they will degenerate.

   b. people will progress at different rates.

   c. you should train at a higher level than you are accustomed to.

   d. you must train an activity to master it.

   e. you should determine your starting points before exercising.

6. The energy system(s) used to produce energy are

   a. the aerobic system.

   b. the oxygen system.

   c. the anaerobic system.

   d. the RPE system.

   e. a and c.

7. Which nutrients provide the most energy for training?

   a. Simple carbohydrates

   b. Complex carbohydrates

   c. Fats

   d. Proteins

   e. Fiber

8. Which of the following represents the ideal meal frequency and nutrient combination?

   a. Three meals per day with protein at every meal

   b. One low-carbohydrate meal per day

   c. Five to six meals per day with high protein at every meal

   d. Eight high-fat meals daily

   e. Six meals daily with balanced protein and carbohydrates at each meal

9. Which of the following combinations are composed of complex carbohydrates?

   a. Brown rice, whole grain pasta, and oatmeal

   b. White rice, cottage cheese, and whole grain pasta

   c. Oatmeal, orange juice, and green beans

   d. Potatoes, honey, and tomatoes

   e. Skim milk, brown rice, and beans

10. Biometric testing will

   a. allow you to customize your training program.

   b. reveal nutritional deficiencies.

   c. provide you with starting points for each exercise.

   d. measure your blood glucose levels.

   e. a and c.

11. The lactate threshold is

   a. the point at which your body transfers from the aerobic to the anaerobic energy system.

   b. your ability to produce power.

   c. your ability to burn fat for extended periods.

   d. your ability to produce speed.

   e. the point at which lactate decreases in the blood.

REFERENCES

1. Nutrition Action Health Letter, (December 2004). Volume 32, Number 10. The Center for Science in the Public Interest. (Washington, D. C.).

2. Glantz, S.A., and W.W. Parmley. Passive and active smoking. A problem for adults. *Circulation* 94(4) (1996): 596–598.

3. American College of Sports Medicine. (2000). *ACSM's Guidelines for Exercise Testing and Prescription*, 6th ed. (Philadelphia: Lippincott Williams & Williams).

4. National Heart, Lung, and Blood Institute. National High Blood Pressure Education Program Working Group report on primary prevention of hypertension. *Archives of Internal Medicine* 153(2) (1993): 186–208.

5. Wang, Y. and Deydoun, M.A. "The Obesity Epidemic in the United States-Gender, Age, Socioeconomic, Racial/Ethnic and Geographic Characteristics: A Systematic Review and Meta-Regression Analysis". *Epidemiologic Reviews* 29, No. 1 (2007): 6–28.

6. Centers for Disease Control and Prevention, National Center for Health Statistics. (2005).

7. American Heart Association. (2006). *Heart and Stroke Facts Statistical Update*. National Center, Dallas, TX.

8. The Canadian Physical Activity, Fitness, & Lifestyle Appraisal: CSEP's Plan for Healthy Active Living. (1996).

9. J. Stevens, J. Cai, E. R. Ramuk, D. F. Williamson, M. J. Thun, and J. L. Wood. "The Effect of Age on the Association Between? Body Mass Index and Mortality". *The New England Journal of Medicine* 338 (1998): 1–7.

10. C. Bouchard, G. A. Bray, and V. S. Hubbard. "Basic and Clinical Aspects of Regional Fat Distribution". *American Journal of Clinical Nutrition* 52 (1990): 946–950.

11. Siff, Mel, et al. (1993). Super training: special strength training for sporting excellence. (South Africa: School of Mechanical Engineering, University of the Witwatersrand).

12. Gledhill, N. and Jammik, VK: Characterization of the Physical Demands of Fire Fighting. *Can J Spt Sci* (1992): 17:3 207–213.

13. Weltman, A., et. al. Exercise training at and above the lactate threshold in previously untrained women. *Int. J. Sports Med.* 13(3) (1992): 257–263.

14. Stone, M.H., et al. Health and performance-related potential of resistance training, *Sports Medicine*, vol. 11(4) (1991): 210–231.

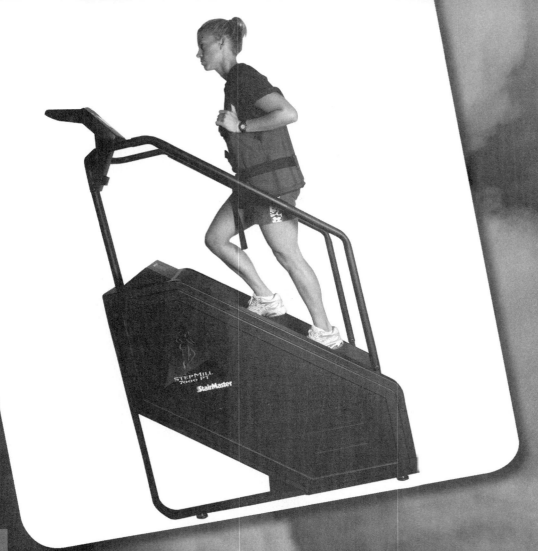

4

Planning Your Workouts

OBJECTIVES

Upon completion of this chapter, the firefighter will be able to

- Understand the role and value of periodization
- Define and describe the elements of the General Adaptation Syndrome
- List five benefits of periodization
- Describe how performance is affected by the timing and intensity of training

- Describe the five phases of a periodization model
- Create a periodized training program using the program design guidelines
- Define the RICE and MICE methods of treating injuries
- List five causes of overtraining

INTRODUCTION

How do you plan workouts? This is a question many firefighters have. They are familiar with many exercises and have used them for years. Yet, the question remains, what exercises are best and how do you design an effective program that addresses the specific needs of firefighters? The ideal program would be one that reduces or eliminates health risk factors, reduces the likelihood of injuries, and increases/maintains one's skills for firefighting.

Fitness program design has both a scientific component and an artistic component. Training principles are the scientific part of fitness, while the artistic part involves blending selected principles into a customized program. While general training principles apply to most people, there is no one single best training program that works for everyone. People have different body types, ages, medical conditions, goals, and abilities. An exercise or technique that works for one individual may not work for another.

PERIODIZATION

Most athletes use planned training strategies designed to prepare them for their specific sport or competition. These programs are collectively known as periodization.

Periodization is a training method that seeks to "peak" an athlete's performance with a competitive event. This is accomplished by changing training intensity and strategically placing maintenance and recovery phases to enhance performance.

In the early 1900's, Canadian scientist Hans Selye developed a theory called the **general adaptation syndrome**, which described an organism's response to stress. He defined a positive adaptation to stress, **eustress**, as being the result of correctly

timed alternation between stress and regeneration. **Distress** is a negative adaptation that occurs when the stimulus is too great or the recovery period too short. Following a positive adaptation to the stress, the organism is capable of doing more work. This enhanced capability is referred to as **supercompensation**.[1,2] From this work, scientists in the former Eastern Bloc countries of the Soviet Union and East Germany evolved the theory of training called periodization. It was not until the later half of the 20th century that the idea of periodizing an athlete's training program became commonly accepted in the United States.[3] Periodization models define the overall training period as being a **macrocycle**, which is divided into smaller phases called **mesocycles**, which are subdivided into weekly **microcycles**.[4]

Periodization and Firefighting Fitness

A periodized training plan will help you plan training sessions in a progressive manner, developing firefighter skills while increasing strength and cardiovascular endurance. It will diminish the chances of overtraining and injury while keeping your workouts interesting and purposeful to prevent boredom. In this chapter, you will learn how to apply this powerful tool to provide maximal benefits and functional improvements for your firefighter career regardless of your age or fitness level, see **Figure 4-1** on the following page. Three different periodization models are presented, enabling you to rotate them in a systematic order to prevent stagnation and maximize training adaptations. Included in each model are planning variations for reducing various health risk factors such as high cholesterol and excess body weight.

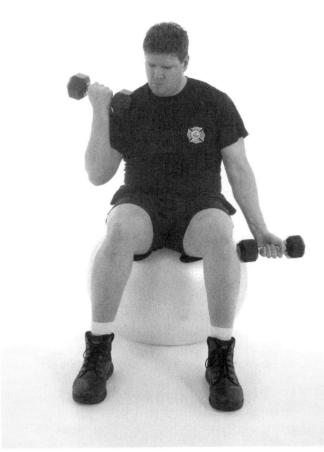

A

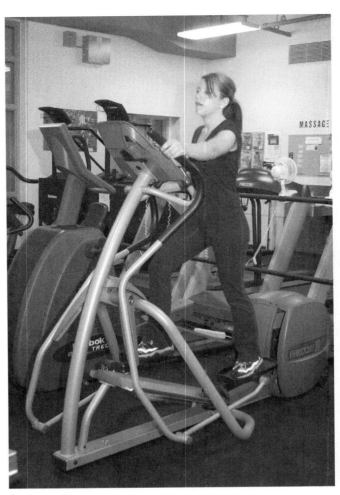

B

FIGURE 4-1 Periodization involves using different training modes to maximize results.

TRAINING PHASES

All periodization models presented here include five phases. Each phase has its own objectives designed to progressively increase your fitness levels and firefighter skills. The phases are

- Base
- Endurance
- Strength
- Power
- Active rest

Base

Objective: Develop a strong cardiovascular and strength base.

Training intensity ranges: Cardiovascular 55% maximum heart rate (MHR), resistance training 15–16 repetitions.

This is a learning phase and a gradual progression is important. If training begins at too high a level, the

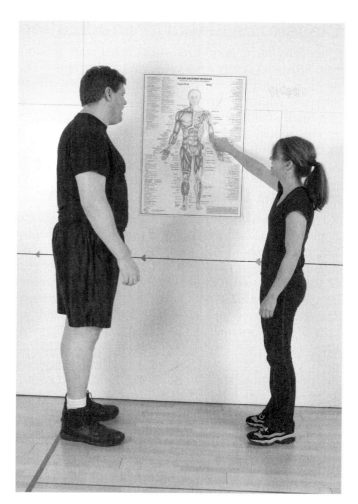

FIGURE 4-2   Planning your program is essential to success.

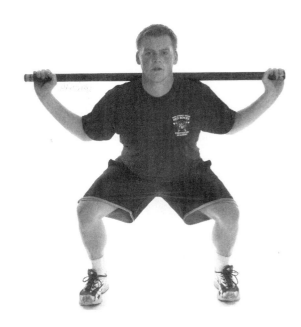

FIGURE 4-3   Developing a strong training base is crucial for goal achievement.

likelihood of illness or injury will increase. The amount of progress made during subsequent phases depends on how solid the training base is, **Figure 4-3**.

Endurance

Objective: Increase the body's ability to maintain exercise for long periods.

Training intensity ranges: Cardiovascular 55–60% MHR, resistance training 12–15 repetitions.

The goal of this phase is to enhance the body's ability to sustain muscular contractions. This conditioning will enhance your ability to perform firefighter duties over an extended period of time.

Strength

Objective: Increase muscular and cardiovascular (anaerobic) strength levels.

Training intensity ranges: Cardiovascular 55–80% MHR, resistance training 6–10 repetitions.

This phase promotes maximal strength development by using basic multi-joint exercises. Longer rest periods are used between strength training sets. Increasing muscular strength is a priority, because as strength decreases so does performance.

Power

Objective: Translate strength into power and train for longer durations at higher intensities.

Training intensity ranges: Cardiovascular 55–90% MHR, resistance training 4–6 repetitions.

Power is the ability to use strength rapidly, and increasing your ability to produce power is crucial to mastering firefighting skills. Raising a ladder, dragging a victim, and climbing stairs all require a firefighter to produce energy in a rapid, forceful manner.

Active Rest

Objective: Allow the body to recover from the training stresses involved in the other phases.

Training intensity ranges: Cardiovascular 55–60% MHR, no resistance training is performed.

Active rest is characterized by activity other than resistance training, such as swimming, hiking or sports activities such as basketball and tennis, see **Figure 4-4** on the following page.[5]

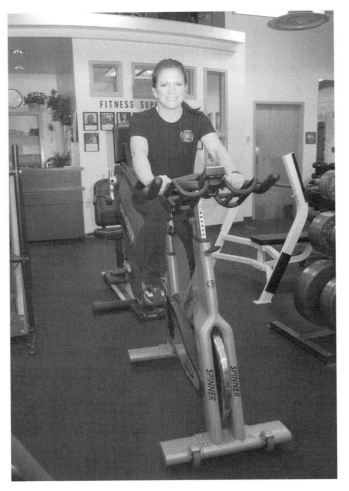

FIGURE 4-4 Including periods of low-intensity training or active rest will reduce your injury risk.

PERIODIZATION MODELS

The three periodization models most commonly used and most extensively researched are classic, or linear, periodization, reverse linear periodization, and undulating periodization.

Classic, or Linear, Periodization

Classic, or linear, periodization is the hallmark training plan most associated with the term periodization. The program's mesocycles progress linearly from a low-intensity endurance phase through a strength phase and finally culminate in a high-intensity power phase.

This model is ideal when training for a fitness test or competition.

Reverse Linear Periodization

Reverse linear periodization takes the classic linear periodization and runs it backward. The reverse linear method starts with the power, or high intensity, phase and progresses to the strength phase. The goal of these first two phases is to build the strength and power to optimize gains in mass or endurance strength. The endurance phase comes last and involves lower intensity (12–15 reps) and higher volume, which is the best prescription for building muscle mass. Being able to lift heavier weight for the desired number of repetitions during the endurance phase can result in significant gains in muscle mass as well as muscle endurance.

Undulating Periodization

Undulating periodization follows a less linear scheme than does the classic or reverse periodization models. Training phases are staggered within each week, with intensity and volume changing from one workout to another. For example, strength workouts might be performed on Monday, endurance workouts performed on Wednesday, and power workouts performed on Friday. The following week, endurance workouts might be performed on Monday, power workouts on Wednesday, and strength workouts on Friday. Over a three-week period each phase has an equal number of workouts.

Periodization Models

	Training Phase				
Model	one	two	three	four	five
Classic	base	endurance	strength	power	active rest
Reverse	base	power	strength	endurance	active rest
Undulating	base	*	*	*	active rest

* Each training phase in the undulating model includes power, strength, and endurance repetition ranges.

CUSTOMIZING PROGRAMS FOR HEALTH RISK FACTORS

Reducing health-risk factors should be the number one goal of program design, **Figure 4-5**.

The first step in reducing risk factors is to see your physician. A physician's clearance and recommendations take precedence over any program design models.

When designing your program, address the risk factors first. Once the risk factor(s) are controlled or eliminated, use the periodization models to enhance your training. Most health-risk factors can be reduced or eliminated by the synergistic effects of good nutrition, cardiovascular exercise, resistance training and stress management.[6] Fitness program modifications for firefighters with increased health risk factors are listed follow.

Exercise Guidelines for Medical Conditions

Coronary artery disease and high cholesterol: To lower total cholesterol, lose weight, and lower your risk for coronary artery disease, stop smoking, exercise regularly, and monitor your nutritional intake closely. Workout sessions should be focused on maximizing calories expended from cardiovascular exercise. Expending 1,000 to 2,000 calories per week is recommended. Do five to seven exercise sessions per week, starting with 20 minutes, building gradually to 60 minutes at a moderate intensity level. No modifications are necessary for resistance training or functional training.

Obesity: The recommendations that apply to lowering cholesterol apply to reducing body weight, with a couple of modifications. Resistance training exercise should start at a base training level of fifteen repetitions for the first two weeks then progress to ten repetitions per set.

The object is to induce as much muscle growth as possible—the more muscle mass the greater the caloric burn even at rest.

Diabetes: Weight control, regular aerobic exercise, good nutrition, and stress reduction can improve insulin sensitivity, sugar utilization, and

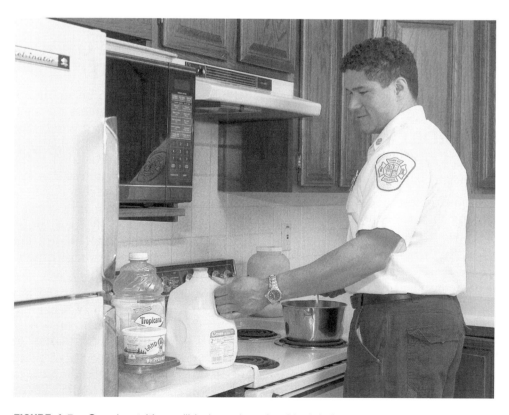

FIGURE 4-5   Good nutrition will help reduce health-risk factors.

generally help control diabetes. Perform four to six sessions of moderate intensity cardiovascular exercise per week, starting with 20 minutes and building gradually to 60 minutes. Resistance training should start with fifteen to twenty repetitions. Individuals with well-controlled diabetes can progress to higher loads and fewer repetitions. Flexibility training should be done a minimum of three sessions per week.

Blood glucose levels should be monitored before and after exercise.

High Blood Pressure: If blood pressure is above 120 systolic and 80 diastolic, an increased risk for coronary artery disease and heart attack is present. Losing weight and exercising are two important steps toward reducing blood pressure. Eating more fruits and vegetables increases potassium intake, and sodium intake should be reduced to less than 2,400 mg per day. Exercise guidelines include performing four to six sessions of long duration, low-intensity cardiovascular exercise per week. Resistance training should be done twice per week, with one set of sixteen to twenty repetitions for each body part until blood pressure normalizes. Avoid holding the breath for extended periods.

Avoid isometric (holding the weight in a stationary position) exercises.

Asthma: Perform four to six sessions of moderate-intensity cardiovascular exercise per week. Divide each session into three or four short segments of 10–15 minutes in duration. Monitor intensity and reduce if any shortness of breath occurs. Start resistance training with high (sixteen to twenty) repetitions. Avoid temperature extremes.

PLANNING GUIDELINES

If you wish to design your own program, use the following guidelines (see Chapter 3 for more detail):

1. Go through the biometric tests and record your results on the planning chart for biometric testing. This will provide you with baseline measures and allow you to set your goals for the entire program.

2. Plan the first phase (base training). Your starting intensities will be determined by the results from your biometric tests.

3. Plan the remaining phases using the principles outlined in the periodization models described in the preceding sections.

4. Evaluate the plan often. If you are meeting your goals and objectives, continue on to the next phase. If your objectives are not being achieved, redesign the next phase and set new goals.

5. If you miss a week of training because of illness or injury, start back where you left off. Do not skip ahead.

6. Monitor your training progress and if overtraining becomes evident, modify the program. In the overall scheme, rest and recovery days are just as important as workout days.

7. As you progress through the training phases, start to develop visual images of yourself executing the exercises with perfect form. Develop focus points and mantras for each exercise.

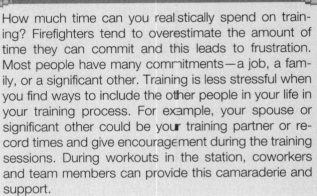

PERFORMANCE POINT

How much time can you realistically spend on training? Firefighters tend to overestimate the amount of time they can commit and this leads to frustration. Most people have many commitments—a job, a family, or a significant other. Training is less stressful when you find ways to include the other people in your life in your training process. For example, your spouse or significant other could be your training partner or record times and give encouragement during the training sessions. During workouts in the station, coworkers and team members can provide this camaraderie and support.

PREPARING FOR A FITNESS TEST

Fire departments often incorporate some form of fitness testing for firefighters on regular schedules. In some cases, firefighters are only required to perform fitness tests at the time they are hired or join a volunteer department. For firefighters who have to maintain a level of fitness for testing, preparation for the test is important for their job and for their livelihood. When you have spent weeks preparing mentally and physically for a firefighter fitness test, what you do in the hours before, during, and after the event can also affect your experience.

Before the test: Make sure you are well-rested. If traveling is necessary for the test, try to arrive a few days early to rest and acclimatize. Drink plenty of water, as travel tends to dehydrate the system. Make sure that anxiety and anticipation about the test do not prevent you from getting plenty of sleep for several nights preceding the test.

Stay with your familiar nutrition program and do not introduce new foods. You do not want any gastric problems on test day.

Scope out the test grounds ahead of time. Set yourself mentally for the arrangement of events. Make adjustments for your mental focus if necessary.

Test day: Time the pre-test meal according to the way you ate meals during training. Stay hydrated. A common mistake is to skip the pretest meal and drink little to avoid frequent trips to the Porta Potty.

Stay focused. Enjoy the day and let it unfold one step at a time. Maintain concentration—don't get caught up in the crowd and what other people are doing.

After the test: Change your clothes, stretch, or get a massage. Relax and enjoy the moment. Rehydrate and refuel.

Don't be alarmed if you experience "post-test depression." Many people liken the feeling to the depression experienced by new mothers.

Relax and enjoy activities with friends.

PERFORMANCE POINT

Working extra hard in the final days before a fitness test drains your energy. You can be rested and mentally ready by doing nothing except for light walking and stretching the last two days before a test. Take your mind off the test by using relaxation and mental focusing techniques.

FITNESS TRAINING CHALLENGES

Delayed-Onset Muscle Soreness

Muscle soreness that occurs 24–48 hours after an activity is called **delayed-onset muscle soreness (DOMS)**. This usually occurs when starting a new activity and is a sign that the body is adapting to a new challenge. The soreness should subside within a few days. The best strategy is to perform active rest (a light activity that involves using the sore muscles); for example, walking and gentle stretching after exercise. All periodization models have built-in rest periods to allow for recovery from DOMS.

SAFETY

Firefighters should consult their personal physicians concerning the use of nonsteroidal anti-inflammatory drugs (NSAIDS) or other treatments for muscle soreness.

Illness

Should you train when you have a cold or fever? Doing a "neck check" is a good idea:

If your symptoms are runny nose, sneezing, or a scratchy throat (above the neck), exercise at a reduced level. If your symptoms are below the neck, such as a chest cold, chills, vomiting, achy muscles, or a fever, you've probably got a more serious viral infection, such as the flu. Exercising intensely in this condition will increase the severity of this illness and can cause extreme complications.

Trying to push past the flu will likely make your condition worse and cause it to last longer. Rest and let your energy reserves fight the illness.

Injuries

Whether a nagging ache or a more serious problem, injuries do not necessarily mean an end to training. Most firefighters experience some type of injury during their career, and proper diagnosis and treatment of an existing injury is critical to maintaining a training schedule. Designing a program that considers past injuries is important, because although the injury has healed, the new tissue will likely never be as strong as the tissue it has replaced.[7]

Acute injuries can be the product of blunt trauma or of overstretching a muscle, joint, or a tendon. Overstretching can cause a tear, sprain, or strain and if left untreated may turn into a chronic condition. Injuries involving pain lasting more than a week, redness, shooting pain, swelling, or a clicking sound in the joints may be an indication of a severe injury that requires a doctor's attention.

Chronic injuries are often the result of overtraining. Repeated bouts of high stress, sudden increases in activity, running on new or uneven surfaces, and inadequate shoe support can cause injuries such as shin splints, plantar faciitis, and achilles tendonitis.

Treating Injuries

The traditional treatment for injuries such as those mentioned above is the use of **RICE:** an acronym for rest, ice, compression, and elevation. As we learn more about the body's own healing mechanisms, we are finding that RICE may not be the best treatment. Immobilizing an injury (unless it's a fracture, torn muscle, or your doctor advises it) restricts blood flow and decreases the temperature of the tissues, which need to be at 100.7 degrees Fahrenheit for the cells to do their job.

Treating injuries by using the **MICE** technique moves the affected area through its functional range

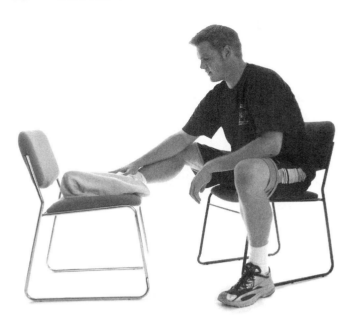

FIGURE 4-6   Using MICE to treat injuries.

of motion, **Figure 4-6**. This increases blood flow to the area, maintaining a healing temperature for the tissues. Guidelines for using MICE are as follows:

■ **Movement:** Slowly move the affected area through its range of motion. Use gentle stretching.

■ **Ice:** Put ice on the injury for 20 minutes, three to four times per day. Place a towel between the skin and the ice so you don't get frostbite. A bag of frozen corn or peas makes a great reusable ice bag.

■ **Compression:** Wrap a towel or ACE bandage around the area. It should be tight enough to support the joint but not too tight. Start wrapping farther away from the heart and apply the bandage upward. Be cautious about sleeping while wearing something that can compromise circulation.

■ **Elevation:** Raise the injured body part so it's slightly higher than your heart, **Figure 4-6**.

PERFORMANCE POINT

Injuries rarely "just happen". Listen to your body and pay attention to warning signs: pain, soreness, aching, and fatigue. Never brush off suspicious symptoms. Instead, make immediate adjustments to your training or seek a professional opinion.

Common Injuries

The following is a list of common injuries that can be experienced during fitness training.

Blisters involve fluid-filled skin that develops from constant exposure to a point of friction. Treatment involves removing the irritation, protecting the affected area, and leaving the skin in place.

A sprain is a complete or partial tear of a ligament, the fibrous connective tissue that binds bones together. Ankle sprains involve swelling and tenderness on the outside of the ankle. Treatment involves using MICE and strengthening the joint when pain and swelling subside.

Plantar fasciitis is a microtearing of the fascia at the bottom of the foot. Common treatment for plantar fasciitis is rest, ice massage, stretching, modifications in training intensity, and strengthening of the muscles of the foot and ankle. Training programs should progress gradually with sudden increases in training intensity being avoided.

A strain is an injury to muscle tissue that is healed with collagen tissue. Stretching and the gradual addition of strengthening exercises are needed to help the collagen tissue form in the proper manner. Treatment involves resting from activity that caused the strain and using MICE on the injured area.

Rotator cuff strain is the overstretching, overexertion, or overuse of the rotator cuff muscles. Rest, stretching, and slowly progressive strengthening exercises are used to return the shoulder to pre-injury function.

Rotator cuff impingement is a common overuse syndrome of the shoulder and is treated by resting the area, stretching, and gradual strengthening exercises such as internal and external rotation, **Figure 4-7**. If treated early, individuals will return to full functional capacity.[8]

Lateral Epicondylitis ("Tennis Elbow") is an overuse injury affecting the outside of the elbow. Repetitive activities involving the wrist, such as playing tennis, carpentry, or pruning shrubs, result in microdamage to the tissue. Cortisone injections and surgery are used when conservative management is not successful.

Lower Back Injuries

Lower back injuries are one of the leading causes of pain and disability for firefighters. Relatively few lower back injuries occur from a single event. The culminating injury event is usually preceded by a history of accumulated trauma produced by the following factors:

■ High repetition lifting of heavy *and* light loads

■ Using improper lifting techniques

■ Not maintaining proper body posture (neutral position) when sitting, standing, and when performing firefighting duties

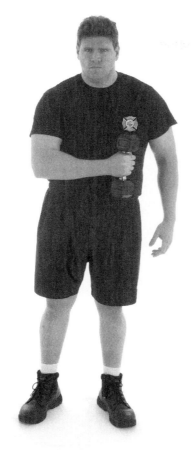

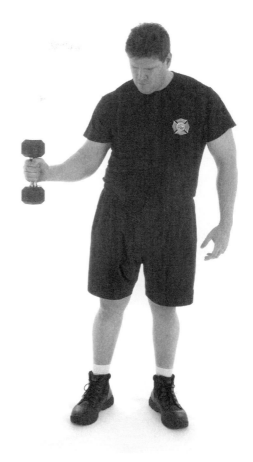

A

B

FIGURE 4-7   Internal and external rotation.

■ Increased stress on the lower back caused by excess abdominal weight

All of these factors act to gradually, but progressively, wear down the supportive structures of the lower back.[9,10]

The Importance of Proper Posture

Firefighters often find themselves in contoured, twisted positions. This is unavoidable and it is unrealistic to expect firefighters to maintain proper posture 100 percent of the time. What is realistic is to minimize these stressful positions and keep the body as fit as possible. A strong core and legs will go a long way in reducing stress to the lower back.

Maintaining a **neutral spine position**, see **Figure 4-8** on the following page, will reduce the risk of many back injuries. A neutral spine position enables a firefighter to apply his or her maximal strength and

will place the least amount of stress or cumulative trauma on the lower back.[9] When the spine is not in a neutral position, such as in a fully flexed or rotated position, the biomechanical or shearing forces are increased dramatically and there is a much greater risk of sustaining an injury.

Lower Back Exercise Recommendations

1. Maintain good cardiovascular fitness.

Mounting evidence supports the role of aerobic exercise in both reducing the incidence of lower back injury and also in the treatment of lower back injuries. The frequency and severity of chronic lower back pain are decreased in individuals who exhibit good cardiovascular fitness, strong abdominal musculature, and good lower back muscle strength.

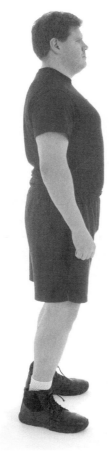

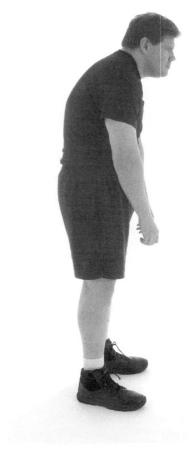

A   B

FIGURE 4-8   (A) Good neutral position for back. (B) Poor neutral position—back is rounded.

2. Keep the body strong, especially the core and legs.

A strong core (abdominal and lower back) and legs will reduce stress on the lower back. Multi-joint exercises such as leg presses, walking lunges, and partial deadlifts build good leg and core strength.

Abdominal exercises should include horizontal side support, **Figure 4-9**. This exercise challenges the lateral obliques without compressing the spine and also activates the quadratus lumborum, which is a significant stabilizer of the spine.[16]

Perform abdominal and lower back exercises later in the day when the fluid level in the discs is better suited to movement.[10] Lower back exercises should be performed with high repetitions.[11]

3. Include flexibility exercises in your training.

Flexibility exercises should include the "cat stretch," **Figure 4-10**, and lower back stretches (knees into chest, spinal twist).

4. Minimize accumulated trauma or stress placed on the lower back.

Avoid prolonged sitting, repetitive bending, vibration, and rounding of the back.

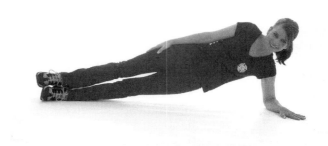

FIGURE 4-9   Horizantal side support.

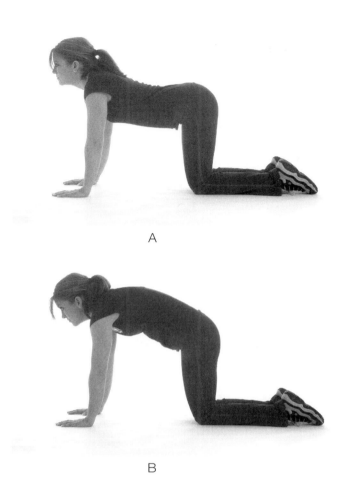

A

B

FIGURE 4-10   Cat stretch.

5. Reduce excess abdominal girth.

Excess weight around the midsection places extraordinary stress on the low back muscles.

Abdominal Belts

The use of abdominal belts (weight training belts) used to be widespread in health clubs and workout facilities. Recently, weight belts have come under scrutiny as to their effectiveness. Wearing a weight belt will tend to increase intra-abdominal pressure and blood pressure. This will enable the lifter to lift slightly more weight than he or she would have without a belt. However, those who have had an injury risk a more severe injury while wearing a belt, and those who have never had a previous back injury appear to have no additional protective benefit from wearing a belt.[12] Ironically, constant use of weight belts will actually weaken the lower back muscles because the belt will "take over" the job of the lower back muscles, thus allowing them to weaken.

Recommendations for weight belt use:

1. Focus on proper body posture when training.

2. If a weight belt is used, use it for the heaviest sets only. Tighten it only when performing the exercise set. Once the set is completed, loosen the belt.

Lower Back Injury Guidelines

Consultation with a doctor or a physical therapist will determine the most appropriate rehabilitative exercises. Patience and compliance are important aspects, as 80 percent of patients who experience lower back pain are pain free within four to six weeks if they stick to their rehabilitation program. Severe lower back pain and injury may take up to three months to resolve.[13]

Treating a lower back injury.

■ Emphasize cardiovascular training at the beginning of a rehabilitation program. Aerobic conditioning produces a much greater rehabilitative effect than strength training.[14] The spine receives its nutrients through the process of diffusion, and cardiovascular exercise is the best mode for accomplishing this.

■ Endurance training should precede specific strengthening exercises in a gradual progressive exercise program. Avoid high impact activities such as jumping. Substitute low- or non-impact exercise such as walking and swimming.

■ Avoid exercises that vertically load the spine, such as shoulder bar presses, squats, bike riding, bent-over rows, and deadlifts.

■ Avoid prolonged sitting, repetitive bending, or vibration. Sitting exercises place more stress on the lower back than standing or lying.

■ Monitor body mechanics and postural position during all activities. Avoid forward flexion and twisting of the spine. Maintaining a neutral position of the spine at all times is crucial.

■ Increase and maintain flexibility in the lower back region. Perform static stretching for the lower back.

■ Reduce excess weight, especially around the midsection.

Recovering from an Injury

One of the five parts of the firefighters' Wellness-Fitness Initiative (WFI) involves rehabilitation from occupational injuries: "Management and labor shall work together to provide a progressive individualized injury/fitness/medical rehabilitation program that shall insure full rehabilitation of any affected uniformed personnel to a safe return to duty status."

NFPA 1500 (Section 8-7.1) states that "It shall be an ongoing objective of the fire department to assist members affected by occupational injuries or illnesses in their rehabilitation and to facilitate their return to full active duty or limited duty where possible." Rehabilitation programs can be in-house or outsourced. Included in these services are physical therapy, work hardening, physical performance assessments, personal training, and an alternate duty program.

It is important for the firefighter to remember that mental training plays a significant role in the healing of the body. How will you react to being injured? Will the experience build you up or tear you down? Top level Olympic athletes use mental imagery techniques to speed up the injury healing process. Kerrin Lee Gartner, Olympic gold medalist for the Canadian women's Alpine ski team, said: "It wasn't the physical recovery but the mental recovery that was the hardest part. It was always important to keep my goals set, to always believe in myself, and to look at the reasons why I was going through these struggles." By relaxing and focusing on specific functions within your own body, you can effect physiological changes in your muscle tension, blood pressure, respiratory rate, blood flow, and body temperature, and even influence your rate of recovery from injury. Visualize the body part you want to influence and then feel the desired change taking place. Use relaxation and mental imagery to recover from injury by visualizing yourself performing firefighter tasks. When you go back to duty, it will be like you never left.

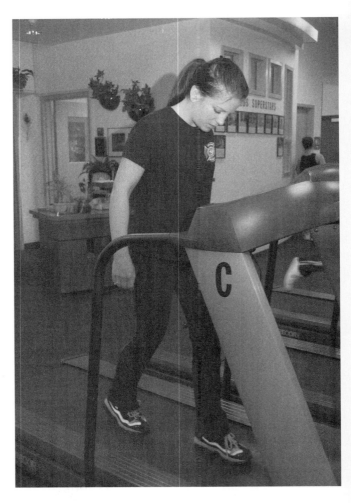

FIGURE 4-11 Overtraining can severely affect your training and firefighter performance.

OVERTRAINING

If training is leaving you more exhausted than energized, it is possible that you are overtraining, **Figure 4-11**. **Overtraining** is decreased work capacity resulting from too little rest or too much training. Excessive training can put your health at risk if adequate rest periods are not built into your program.

Prevention is the best strategy. This involves planning out a program tailor-made to fit your goals and capabilities. It also involves "listening to your body": how you feel during training and when performing firefighter duties. If a workout of similar intensity feels harder or takes longer to recover from, you may be headed to a state of overtraining. Recovery from overtraining usually takes about four to six weeks.

Symptoms of overtraining include:

- Decreased performance
- Agitation, moodiness, irritability, or lack of concentration
- Excessive fatigue
- Increased perceived effort during workouts
- Chronic or nagging muscle aches or joint pain
- Frequent illnesses and upper-respiratory tract infections
- Insomnia or restless sleep
- Loss of appetite and excessive weight loss
- Elevated resting heart rate
- Menstrual cycle disturbances in women
- Muscle or joint pain that lingers longer than 48 hours

CASE STUDIES
Using Periodization to Achieve Fitness Goals

Firefighters Jennifer and Art developed the following training goals after undergoing biometric testing to determine baseline measurements and starting points.

Case Study One: Firefighter Jennifer

Biometric Testing/Health Screening

Body Weight: 160 pounds

Height: Five foot six inches

Total Cholesterol: 240 mg/DL (high)

Body Fat Percentage: 25%

1.5 mile run time: 16:11 (minutes:seconds)

Bench Press test: 55 pounds for one repetition (poor)

Dummy Drag test: Failed to complete

pull-ups: 2 reps

push-ups (full body): 5 reps

Goals

Jennifer set three specific goals:

Goal one: Decrease her time in the mile and one-half run from 16:11 minutes to 12:00 minutes

Objective: Develop a progressive running schedule.

Goal two: Decrease her body fat level from 25 percent to 19 percent

Objective: Consult with a registered dietitian to develop a nutritional program for weight and fat loss.

Goal three: Increase her upper body strength

Objective: Develop a progressive strength training schedule.

Skill Learning

Jennifer consulted with a nationally certified personal trainer when developing her program.

Program Plan

Jennifer decided to use a reverse linear periodization schedule for both her cardiovascular and resistance training programs. Her goals are interdependent and her efforts will act synergistically to aid the completion of each goal. The improvement in her nutritional program will help to lower her running time and reduce her body fat levels. The conditioning from the running and strength training programs will increase her metabolism and help to lower her body fat. Likewise, a reduction in her body fat level will enhance her running ability.

Jennifer's program
Resistance training

To maximize her training time, Jennifer will use one multi-joint exercise per body part. Her training will be divided into two three-month mesocycles. Exercises for each body part will be divided into A and B categories: the A exercises will be used for the first three-month mesocycle and the B exercises used for the second three-month mesocycle. She will superset her exercises during the endurance phase of each mesocycle. This will train her system to tolerate large amounts of lactic acid buildup, increasing her ability to maintain a high performance level while in a fatigued state.

A exercises:

upper body	lower body and shoulders
barbell bench press	leg press
dumbbell row	seated calf-raise
bench dip	walking lunge
EZ bar curl	leg press calf-raise dumbbell press

B exercises:

upper body	lower body and shoulders
incline dumbbell press	split squat
seated row	seated calf-raise
closed-grip press	walking lunge
dumbbell curl	leg press calf machine shoulder press

Using Periodization to Achieve Fitness Goals

Resistance training program

Sets: three per exercise
Repetitions per set

Day	Mon	Tue	Thur	Fri
Body parts	upper body	lower body	upper body	lower body
Week 1	15	15	15	15
Week 2	6–8	6–8	6–8	6–8
Week 3	10–12	10–12	10–12	10–12
Week 4	12–15	12–15	12–15	12–15
Week 5	Active rest–cardio and stretching only			

Cardiovascular training

Jennifer will use a combination of the stepmill, treadmill, or outside running and cycle class or outside cycling. The cycle workouts are non-impact and will give her a cardiovascular workout without stressing the joints.

Week 2 is a high-intensity week with two lower-intensity days mixed in. The low-intensity workouts are done on Tuesdays and Thursdays to allow the heart to rest between the high-intensity sessions.

Workout	minutes/intensity			
Week/day	Mon	Wed	Thr	Sat
Week 1	30/low	40/low	45/low	45/low
Week 2	30/mod	30/high	35/low	45/high
Week 3	30/mod	40/mod	45/mod	30/mod
Week 4	40/low	60/low	40/low	60/low
Week 5	60/low	45/low	60/low	50/low

Functional training

Workout	Tue	Wed	Thur	Sat
Exercises				
Week 1	basic	basic	basic	basic
Sets/reps	1/10	1/10	1/10	1/10
Week 2-4	basic	advanced	basic	advanced
Sets/reps	1/10	1/15	2/10	2/20
Week 5	Active rest-cardio and stretching only			

Functional training exercises:

Tuesday	Thursday
split squat	floor crunch
walking lunge	fit ball crunch with medicine ball
diagonal crunch	Russian twist on fit ball with medicine ball
floor plank	BOSU plank
fit ball hyperextension	BOSU push-up

BOSU standing and squatting
BOSU one-leg balance

Flexibility training

Workout	Mon	Wed	Thur	Sat
Stretches	Sets/duration (seconds)			
Week 1	1/15	1/15	1/15	1/15
Week 2–5	1/15	2/20	1/15	2/20

Flexibility exercises:

Duration: hold each stretch 20–30 seconds	
Repetitions: Perform each stretch one time	
Seated hamstring stretch	Standing calf-stretch, straight leg
Seated inner thigh stretch	Standing calf-stretch, bent leg
Lying hip stretch	Hip flexor stretch
Standing quadriceps stretch	Lying lower back
Lying spinal twist	

Program results

Jennifer's program results are listed below:

	Starting	Ending
Goal 1: 1½ miles run time (minutes)	16:11	10:55
Goal 2: Body fat reduction	25%	18%
Goal 3: Upper body strength increase:		
pull-ups	2 reps	5 reps
push-ups (full body)	5 reps	15 reps

Using Periodization to Achieve Fitness Goals

Jennifer achieved her goals. She also reduced her body weight by 10 pounds, which consisted of a loss of 12 pounds of fat and an increase of 2 pounds of muscle.

As she progressed through the program, the improvement in her goals blended synergistically. The reduction in her body weight aided her run time and pull-up strength. Her improvement in the mile and one-half run time facilitated the reduction in body fat level.

After taking a week off, Jennifer set new goals and developed a new training program using several new exercises, which will include yoga and different functional training exercises.

Case Study Two: Firefighter Art

Goals

Art set three specific goals:

Goal One: Reduce his blood pressure from 160/100 to 120/80

Objective: Develop a training plan that will balance cardiovascular, weight training, and relaxation techniques.

Goal Two: Reduce his body weight from 260 pounds to 200 pounds

Objective: Consult with a registered dietician to develop a nutritional plan

Goal Three: Reduce his total cholesterol reading from 320 mg/dL to 200 mg/dL

Objective: Develop a cardiovascular training program that will expend 1,500 calories per week.

Skill Learning

Art consulted with a nationally certified personal trainer for help in designing his training program.

Program Plan

Resistance training program

Art decided to train with another firefighter who was also trying to lose weight. Training with a partner enabled Art to exercise with a spotter, which enabled him to safely complete the heavier strength training sets. Art and his partner used the mental training technique of visualization, encouraging each other to visualize completing each exercise with perfect execution.

Art chose a linear periodization model with three mesocycles of five weeks each.

Because cardiovascular training will have the greatest influence on achieving his goals, he will limit his resistance training to two days per week—one lower body day and one upper body day. He will use one multi-joint exercise per body part.

Weight training exercises:

upper body	lower body
incline dumbbell bench press	leg press
dumbbell row	seated calf-raise
closed-grip press	walking lunge
EZ bar curl	leg press calf-raise
Machine shoulder press	

Resistance training mesocycle:
Sets: 3 per exercise

Repetitions per set

Day	Training phase	Mon	Thur
Body parts		upper body	lower body
Week 1	Base	15	15
Week 2	Endurance	12–15	12–15
Week 3	Strength	10–12	10–12
Week 4	Power	6–8	6–8
Week 5	Active rest–cardiovascular training and stretching only		

Cardiovascular training program

Art's trainer substituted stationary bike riding and treadmill walking on an incline instead of hill and flat running. Art noticed that his back and knees stopped aching and his energy level increased.

Using Periodization to Achieve Fitness Goals

Week 4 is a high-intensity, or power-training, week with two lower-intensity days mixed in. The low-intensity-workouts are done on Wednesdays and Saturdays to allow the heart to rest between the high-intensity sessions.

Cardiovascular training mesocycle:

		minutes/intensity		
Workout	Mon	Wed	Thur	Sat
Week 1	30/low	40/low	45/low	45/low
Week 2	30/mod	30/low	35/mod	45/low
Week 3	30/mod	40/mod	45/mod	30/mod
Week 4	40/high	60/low	40/high	60/low
Week 5	60/low	45/low	60/low	50/low

Functional training program

Because his goals are involved health improvement, Art performed only a limited amount of functional training exercises:

Monday exercises:	fit ball crunch with medicine ball and fit ball hyperextension
Thursday exercises:	floor crunch, floor plank and split squat
Sets/reps	
Week 1	1/10
Week 2–4	1/15
Week 5	Active rest–cardio and stretching only

Flexibility program

While stretching after each workout, Art and his partner reviewed the exercises completed and provided each other with feedback about their performance. The flexibility exercises chosen emphasized lower back stretching and were performed after each workout for the duration of his program.

Flexibility exercises:

Seated hamstring stretch	Seated inner thigh stretch
Lying hip stretch	Lying lower back
Lying spinal twist	

Art and his partner also attended a yoga class on Tuesdays.

Feedback

A primary care physician measured Art's blood pressure, body weight and waist.

Art and his training partner kept detailed training logs of their exercise sessions. They had their blood pressure and body weight measured every two weeks.

Program results

Art's program results are listed below:

	Starting	Ending
Goal 1: Blood pressure reduction	160/100	130/80
Goal 2: Bodyweight reduction	260 lbs	208 lbs
Goal 3: Cholesterol reduction	320 mg/dL	215 mg/dL

Although Art fell short of achieving his goals, his progress was very good. The momentum gained in his first training schedule will serve him well. To celebrate his progress, his wife treated him to dinner on the last evening of the program. After taking a week off, he developed a new training schedule using an undulating periodization schedule.

Case Study Three: Firefighter Joe

Health Screening and Biometric Testing

Age: 43

Height: 6'0"

Weight: 230 pounds

Cholesterol: 255 mg/dL

Waist measurement: 41 inches

Lower back injury

Goals

Joe's goals included reducing his body weight by 40 pounds, reducing his cholesterol to 190 mg/dL, and increasing his lower back strength. His doctor said that his waist measurement of 41 inches was placing a lot of stress on his lower back.

Skill Learning

Joe hired a certified personal trainer to design and coach him through the first seven weeks of his program.

Using Periodization to Achieve Fitness Goals

Program Plan

Using the advice of his trainer, Joe decided to use an undulating periodization program for his resistance training but not to use a periodized program for his cardiovascular exercise. Instead, he will maintain a high volume of cardiovascular training throughout the duration of the program in an effort to reduce his cholesterol levels and body weight. In addition, Joe will include functional exercises to increase the strength and flexibility of his lower back.

Cardiovascular program

Joe will use treadmill walking at medium intensity for 40–60 minutes, for five to six days per week. Walking is easier on the lower back, and a medium intensity level will enable Joe to complete 60 minutes. Joe will also bike and hike outside when the weather permits.

Mondays and Thursdays							
Week	1	2	3	4	5	6	7
Monday (sets/reps)	2/16	2/8	2/6	2/14	2/10	2/8	active rest
Thursday (sets/reps)	2/16	2/12	2/10	2/8	2/6	2/12	active rest

Resistance training program

Joe will use six multi-joint exercises and perform them in the following order (largest muscle groups to smaller groups):

1. Leg press
2. Dumbbell bench press
3. Lat pull-down
4. Closed-grip press
5. Seated dumbbell curl
6. Bodyweight walking lunge

No overhead pressing movements are included because of the stress they place on the lower back. Dumbell lateral raises will be included starting with the tenth week, or second macrocycle.

Functional/flexibility program

Joe will focus on three functional exercises designed to strengthen his lower back:

- Horizontal side support
- Superman exercise: arms and legs elevated while lying face down
- Contra-laterals: opposite arm and leg elevated while lying face down

He will perform these exercises every workout, immediately after his abdominal training. Additionally, he will perform lower back and hip stretches after all workouts.

Feedback

Joe will receive feedback from his workout records and weekly weigh-ins. He will visit his doctor on the seventh week for blood panel and blood pressure testing. He will use these results to set new goals and design a second program, or mesocycle, which will start in the eighth week.

Case Study Four: Firefighter Cindy

Health Screening and Biometric Testing

Age: 26

Height: 5'8"

Weight: 130 pounds

All biometric tests are normal except upper body strength, which is low.

Goals

Cindy's goal is to pass a firefighter fitness test that is being held in nine weeks.

Cindy set two objectives for this goal. She will increase her upper body strength and cardiovascular capacity to levels that will meet the demands of the test. Cindy will also include exercises for functional flexibility training.

Skill Learning

Cindy bought a book on passing the firefighter fitness test and also learned about the test requirements from other firefighters who have passed it.

Program Plan

Cindy will use a linear (classic) periodization model for both her cardiovascular and strength programs. This will enable her to be in peak condition for the test.

Using Periodization to Achieve Fitness Goals

Resistance training program

Mondays and Thursdays					
	week 1–2	week 3–4	week 5–6	week 7–8	week 9
Training phase	base	endurance	strength	power	test
Sets/reps	2/16	2/15	3/10	3/6-8	n/a

She will use supersets (performing two exercises back-to-back without resting) to save time and also to keep her heart rate elevated. This will produce a training effect that is similar to the fitness test. The program combines seven multi-joint exercises with two supporting exercises and is performed in the following order:

1. Leg press and seated calf-raise superset
2. Dumbbell bench press and dumbbell row superset
3. Closed-grip press and lat pull-down superset
4. Standing EZ bar curl and seated dumbbell shoulder press superset
5. Walking lunge with dumbbells

Cardiovascular training program:

Tuesdays and Fridays

Cindy will use a stepmill, a treadmill, and outside running for her cardiovascular training. She will use a weight vest when training on the stepmill in order to simulate the test event. Treadmill walking will be done at high-intensity intervals for the strength and power phases and at a constant speed and elevation for the base and endurance phases. Outside running will be done on mostly flat ground during the base and endurance phases, with hill running incorporated during the strength and power phases.

Cardiovascular Training Levels

	week 1–2	week 3–4	week 5–6	week 7–8	week 9
Training phase	base	endurance	strength	power test	
Intensity	low	low/medium	medium/high	high	

Tuesday workouts				
Treadmill	30 min.	30 min.	20 min.	20 min.
Stepmill	10 min.	10 min.*	5 min.*	

Friday workouts				
Outside running	30 min.	30 min.	20 min.	20 min.
Stepmill	10 min.	10 min.*	5 min.*	

* with weight vest

Functional/Flexibility Plan:

Wednesdays: Cindy will use a training circuit that will be an actual or close simulation of each event in the test. Wednesdays and Saturdays: Cindy will perform core strengthening exercises using a fit ball and a medicine ball, as follows:

- Basic crunch
- Russian twist
- Hyperextension
- Plank with feet elevated on the Fit Ball
- Push-ups with feet elevated on the Fit Ball, progressing to push-ups with one hand on the medicine ball

She will perform lower back, hip flexor, and inner thigh stretches after all workouts.

Active Rest

Cindy will not train on the two days prior to the test to ensure that she is well-rested.

Feedback

Cindy will receive feedback on her test time by taking a trial run on the test course. Feedback will also be generated from her workout records and extra training on the dummy drag. For the circuit training, she will use a stopwatch and also have other firefighters watch her performance.

Using Periodization to Achieve Fitness Goals

Case Study Five: Firefighter Mike

Health Screening and Biometric Testing

Age: 32

Height: 5'10"

Weight: 195 pounds

Cholesterol: 205 mg/dL

Blood pressure: 130/85

Body fat percentage: 26%

Goals

Mike's goals are to reduce his slightly elevated cholesterol and blood pressure levels. His biggest goal is to reduce his body fat level.

Skill Learning

Mike consulted with the department's certified personal trainer for guidance in developing a training program and learning proper exercise technique.

Program Plan

Mike will be using a reverse periodization program for his resistance and cardiovascular training. He felt that the reverse model would result in greater increases in muscle mass. He will exercise with two other firefighters.

Cardiovascular program

Mike will perform three cardiovascular workouts per week. On Mondays and Fridays he will exercise at a low intensity using a bike or treadmill. On Wednesdays he will alternate using the treadmill and stepmill to perform high-intensity intervals. He will walk and run on the treadmill and use a weight vest when on the stepmill. For his active rest phase he will use the bike.

	week 1–2	week 3–4	week 5–6	week 7–8	week 9
Training phase	base	power	strength	endurance	rest

Wednesday

Intensity	low	high	medium/high	low	low
Treadmill/Step Mill	30 min	.30 min.	20 min.	20 min	
Bike					40 min.

Monday and Friday

Intensity	low	low	low	low	low
Treadmill or bike	40 min.	40 min.	40 min.	40 min	30 min.

Resistance training program:

Tuesdays, Thursdays, and Saturdays

	week 1–2	week 3–4	week 5–6	week 7–8	week 9
Training phase	base	power	strength	endurance rest	
Sets/reps	2/16	3/6	2/8-10	2/14	

Mike will use six multi-joint exercises and perform them in the following order (largest muscle groups to smaller groups):

Workout A: Legs and shoulders

1. Leg press
2. Seated calf-raise
3. Dumbbell walking lunge
4. Dumbbell shoulder press
5. Leg press calf-raise
6. Dumbbell lateral raise

Workout B: Upper body

1. Barbell bench press
2. Dumbbell row
3. Closed-grip press
4. Dumbbell curl
5. Front lat pull-down
6. Overhead rope extension

CASE STUDIES
Using Periodization to Achieve Fitness Goals

Functional/flexibility program

Mike will use a stability ball, a medicine ball, and a BOSU for his core training.

He will use the medicine ball when performing crunches and he will do Russian twists, hyperextensions, and reverse hyperextensions on the stability ball. Planks and push-ups will be performed using the flat side of the BOSU. He will use a slant board to perform lower abdominal work, including hip thrusts and leg drops.

Flexibility work will include quadriceps, hamstrings, lower back, inner thigh, and hip stretches after all workouts.

Feedback

Mike will receive feedback from his workout records and weekly weigh-ins. He will visit his doctor in the ninth week for blood panel and blood pressure testing. He will use these results to set new goals and design a second program, or mesocycle, which will start in the tenth week.

Guidelines for Avoiding Overtraining

1. Make sure you are getting the nutrients to support your training. Eat within 15 to 30 minutes after each training session. Adequate amounts of complex carbohydrates are essential to meet the increased demands placed on your system.

2. Rest, active or passive, is probably the most important strategy. Take at least one rest day per week and additional days if needed.

3. If you are returning from an injury or a short training break, resume the program where you left off. Do not skip ahead a week to make up for lost time. If you miss three to four weeks, start back at a base training phase. You will need to recondition your joints and the affected muscle area.

4. Keeping detailed training records. Individuals vary in their ability to handle different training volumes. You can pinpoint "break points," or what training volumes may produce overtraining for you.

5. Check your pulse for 60 seconds before getting out of bed. If it is five beats higher than normal, you're due for a rest day.

6. Increase your sleep time. This is when recuperation and growth take place.

7. Post-workout ice baths and sports massages improve circulation and flush out waste products, reducing inflammation and soreness.

8. Psychological stress may be additive to the physical stress of training. Psychological stressors may include work, family, competition, travel, and other life stressors. If external personal life stressors are high, reduce your training load. [15]

CHAPTER SUMMARY

Planning an individualized training program is crucial to achieving fitness goals. An ideal way to accomplish this is to use the periodization training model, which strategically changes training intensity, maintenance, and recovery phases.

Periodization is based upon the General Adaptation Syndrome, which states that properly timed stress, or eustress, will produce a supercompensation effect and thus improve performance. Periodized programs have been shown to reduce injuries, prevent overtraining, and produce better results than nonperiodized ones.

Periodization models are divided into training phases. The entire training period is called a macrocycle. Macrocycles are divided into smaller phases of four to six weeks, called mesocycles, which are subdivided into weekly microcycles. Program macrocycles can progress from low to high intensity, high to low intensity, or mix high and low intensities within the same microcycles.

The traditional or linear periodization model consists of four phases of increasing intensity. The first phase is base training, which builds a foundation for the higher intensity training found in the following phases. Fitness testing is done during this phase to determine starting points for all exercises. Phase two focuses on developing strength and endurance by increasing training intensity. Phase three integrates strength and endurance to produce power—the ability to apply strength rapidly. This enables firefighters to maintain their performance for long durations during an emergency. Phase four focuses on active rest to allow the body to rest and prepare for the next mesocycle. Goals are evaluated and reset if necessary at the end of each phase.

Reverse linear periodization reverses the training progression of the linear model. After a short base training microcycle, the program starts with power or high intensity training phase and progresses to the endurance phase. The goal of this model is to build the strength and power to optimize gains in mass or endurance in the last phase.

Undulating periodization follows a less linear scheme than does the classic or reverse periodization models. Training phases are staggered within each week, with intensity and volume changing from one workout to another. Some studies have shown that the undulating model produces superior results compared to traditional or reverse periodization models.

Obstacles such as muscle soreness, injuries, and overtraining sometimes do appear but they do not necessarily mean an end to training if handled correctly.

Muscle soreness that usually subsides within two days after undertaking a new activity is called delayed-onset muscle soreness (DOMS). It is not a serious condition and is best treated by low-intensity activity involving the affected areas. Injuries requiring a doctor's attention include acute injuries, which can be the result of overstretching or blunt trauma, and chronic injuries, which usually result from overtraining. The recommended method of treating injuries is called MICE, an acronym for gentle movement, ice, compression, and elevation. MICE will enhance the body's natural healing mechanisms by promoting blood flow to the affected area(s).

Overtraining is best treated by increasing rest days and ensuring nutrition is adequate to handle the increased demands of training. Monitoring of the training program will reduce the likelihood of overtraining and injuries.

KEY TERMS

Classic or linear periodization   A training method that progresses from low to high intensity exercises.

Delayed-onset muscle soreness (DOMS)   Muscle soreness that occurs 24 to 48 hours after an activity.

Distress   A negative adaptation to stress, resulting when there is too great a stimulus and/or too little regeneration.

Eustress   A positive adaptation to stress, resulting from correctly timed alternation between stress and regeneration.

General adaptation syndrome (GAS)   An organism's response to stress. Positive adaptation to stress is called eustress, being the result of correctly timed alternation between stress and regeneration. Too great a stimulus and /or too little regeneration results in a negative adaptation, or distress.

Macrocycle   An overall training period.

Mesocycle   A major training phase within a macrocycle, usually four to six weeks in length.

MICE   A method of treating injuries, an acronym for movement, ice, compression, and elevation.

Microcycle   A short period of training usually lasting about one week.

Neutral spine position   The neutral position of the spine is the strongest, least stressful position for the body. When an individual's posture is optimal, the head is up, the eyes are looking straight forward, the chest is out, and the lower back has a normal inward curve and the upper back has a normal outward curve.

Overtraining   Decreased work capacity resulting from too little rest or too much training.

Periodization   A training method that seeks to optimize fitness program effectiveness. This is accomplished by changing training intensity and strategically placing maintenance and recovery phases.

Reverse linear periodization   A training method that progresses from high intensity to low intensity exercise.

Supercompensation   An enhanced capability following a positive adaptation to the stress, when the organism is capable of doing more work.

Undulating periodization   A training method that incorporates mixtures of high, medium and low intensities in each training week.

CHECK YOUR LEARNING

1. The concept "supercompensation" refers to
   a. working hard right up to test day.
   b. adapting to training demands.
   c. having someone train with you.
   d. increasing your energy by "carb loading."
2. Benefits of periodization include
   a. enabling you to be at peak performance for a firefighter fitness test.
   b. planning out training.
   c. avoiding injuries.
   d. all of the above.
3. All of the following are components of the General Adaptation Syndrome except
   a. eustress.
   b. maintenance.
   c. supercompensation.
   d. distress.
4. A good treatment for overtraining is to
   a. increase your protein intake and decrease your carbohydrate intake.
   b. take hot showers.
   c. get post-workout massages.
   d. decrease your rest days.
5. Linear periodization phase four training involves
   a. developing peak power.
   b. perfecting skills.
   c. utilizing active rest.
   d. all of the above.
6. Delayed-onset muscle soreness is caused by
   a. overstretching a muscle.
   b. warming up too long.
   c. keeping training intensity constant.
   d. starting new training methods.
7. In physical training, the concept of power refers to
   a. the ability to lift a great amount of weight.
   b. the ability to lift a heavy weight several times.
   c. the ability to train for extended periods.
   d. the ability to use strength rapidly.
8. If your preparation time is limited when training for a fitness test, which two training phases should you focus on?
   a. phases one and three.
   b. phases one and four.
   c. phases two and four.
   d. phases two and three.
9. Linear, or classic, periodization involves
   a. starting with higher repetitions and lower weights, then reducing the repetitions and raising the weights stage-by-stage, every few weeks.
   b. changing the focus from session to session.
   c. sport-specific training.
   d. alternating weight training and plyometrics.
10. Nonlinear, or undulating, periodization involves
    a. increasing intensity in a gradual manner.
    b. changing intensity from session to session.
    c. athletic training drills only.
    d. alternating standing, jumping, and hopping exercises.

REFERENCES

1. Zatsiorsky, V. M. (1995). Science and Practice of Strength Training. Champaign, IL: Human Kinetics.
2. Bompa, T. O. (1999). Periodization: Theory and Methodology of Training. Champaign, IL: Human Kinetics.
3. Lydiard, A., & Gilmour, G. (1978). Running the Lydiard Way. (Mountain View, CA: World Publications). Cited in T.D. Noakes. (1991). Love of Running (155, 157, 209). (Champaign, IL: Leisure Press).
4. Willoughby, D.S. The effects of mesocycle-length weight training programs involving periodization and partially equated volumes on upper and lower body strength. *Journal of Strength and Conditioning Research* 7(1) (1993): 2–8.
5. American College of Sports Medicine (ACSM). (2006). *ACSM's Guidelines for Exercise Testing and Prescription* (7th ed.). Baltimore: Lippincott Williams & Wilkins.
6. Slentz, C.A., et al. Effects of the amount of exercise on body weight, body composition, and measures of central obesity: STRIDE-a randomized controlled study. *Archives of Internal Medicine* 164(1) (2004): 31–39.
7. Leadbetter, W.B. *Cell-matrix response in tendon injuries. Clinics in Sports Medicine* 11(3) (1992): 533–578.
8. Jobe, F. W., & Pink, M. (1993). Classification and treatment of shoulder dysfunction in the overhead athlete. *Journal of Orthopedic and Sports Physical Therapy*, 18, 2, 427–432.
9. McGill SM. ISB Keynote Lecture-The biomechanics of low back injury: Implications on current practice in industry and the clinic. *J Biomech* 30 (1997): 465–475.
10. Adams MA, Dolan P. Recent advances in lumbar spine mechanics and their clinical significance. *Clin Biomech* 10 (1995): 3–19.

11. Potvin JR, Norman RW. Can fatigue compromise lifting safety? : Proc. NACOB II. The Second North American congress on Biomechanics. (August 24–28 1992): 513–514.

12. McGill SM. Abdominal Belts in industry: A position paper on their assets, liabilities and use. Am Ind Hyg Assoc J 54 (1993): 752–754. (ref 46) Nutter P. Aerobic exercise in the treatment and prevention of low back pain. Occup Med 3 (1988):137–145.

13. Manniche C, Hesselsoe G, Bentxen L, et al. Clinical trial of intensive muscle training for chronic low back pain. *Lancet* 24 (1988): 1473–1476.

14. Cady LD, Bischoff DP, O'Connell ER, et al. Strength and fitness and subsequent back injuries in firefighters. J Occup Med 21(4) (1979): 269–272.

15. Armstrong, L. E., and J.L. VanHeest. The unknown mechanism of the overtraining syndrome. *Sports Med*. 32 (2002): 185–209.

16. McGill SM, Juker D, Kropf P. Quantitative intramuscular myoelectric activity of quadratus lumborum during a wide variety of tasks. Clin Biomech 11(3) (1996): 170–172.

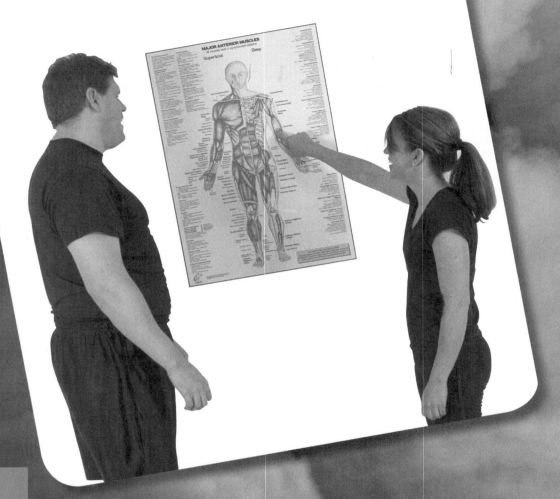

5

Creating a Healthy Culture

OBJECTIVES

Upon completion of this chapter, the firefighter will be able to

- Recognize the influence that a department's culture has on a firefighter's health
- Learn the five steps to creating a healthy fire department culture
- List and describe the five stages in the Stages of Change model
- Understand the importance of involving the entire staff in developing a cultural-change plan
- Analyze a fire department's culture and how it affects each firefighter's fitness and health levels

- Analyze an individual's readiness to change by using the Stages of Change model
- Plan equipment purchases and design an exercise area
- List the advantages of various types of cardiovascular equipment
- Describe the concepts and usefulness of brainstorming and the nominal group technique in generating ideas for cultural change

INTRODUCTION

A healthy, innovative, and productive **culture** is one that energizes the workforce through multiple sources: physical, emotional, intellectual, and spiritual. Fire chiefs, company officers, and individual firefighters must realize the influence that their departmental cultural has on each firefighter's health. The only way firefighters can improve and maintain their health is to have a supportive culture—a culture that promotes health, innovation, and productivity, **Figure 5-1**.

If you ask somebody to swim in a pool and create a current against them, most people are just not going to be successful in reaching the other end of the pool. A workplace culture that does not support firefighters' health is like making them swim upstream, against the current; change the culture to one that encourages positive health practices and innovation and you make it easy for them to flow downstream. That makes all the difference.

Changing the culture of a fire department from an "unhealthy" one to a "healthy one" can seem like an overwhelming task. But by following the change process presented below you can be confident that you have covered all the key areas that are involved in changing your departmental culture to a healthier one.

CULTURAL CHANGE PROCESS
Step 1: Develop a Vision of Where You Want to Be

Begin with a vision of what you want the culture to look like when you finish with the change process. Conduct meetings and distribute surveys to gather input from every firefighter and all areas of the department. Once all the input has been gathered, create a vision statement of what the ideal fitness and health culture would look like.

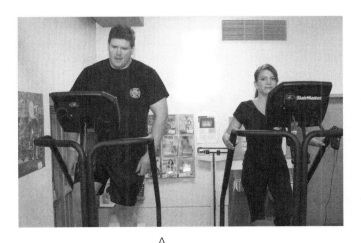

A

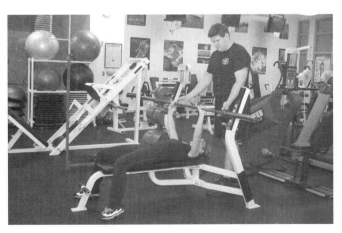

B

FIGURE 5-1   A healthy work culture develops and supports each firefighter's teamwork and job skills.

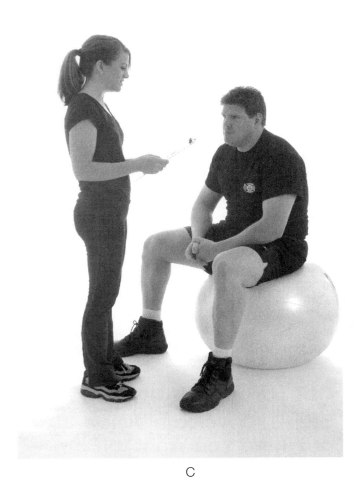

C

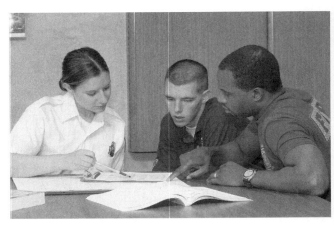

D

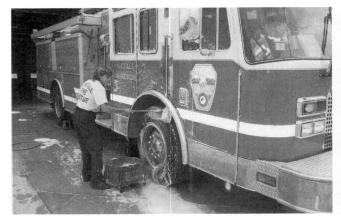

E

FIGURE 5-1 Continued.

Key questions to address:

- What do you want to create for the future? Do you want exercise time, facilities, healthy nutritional offerings, and so on?
- What are the five most important fitness and health values you would like to see represented in your culture?
- Are these values represented in your current culture? If not, why not?
- If they are so important, why are you not attaining these values?

Step 2: Find Out Where You Are Now

This step involves determining how important fitness and health are currently within the department. How strong are the fitness norms and values and are they getting better or getting worse?

Assess the firefighters' perceptions of the current culture and how it enhances or detracts from their ability to maintain their health and fitness. Formal and informal meetings with each member of the department and gathering data through surveys are two ways to determine each member's perceptions.

It is crucial to determine:

- How important are health and fitness to each firefighter?
- How committed is the department to employee fitness and health?
- Does the present departmental culture help or impede the firefighters' ability to maintain their fitness and health?
- Is the department getting closer to or moving away from a fitness culture?

Step 3: Develop Plans to Change the Departmental Culture

Firefighters can create the kind of culture they want if they have a chance to be involved in its creation. Involve the entire staff in developing plans that will enable firefighters to make the necessary changes to improve their health and fitness levels, **Figure 5-2**.

First, share the results from the first two steps with the entire department. The truth is, the results are nothing to be scared of, and if you communicate them to firefighters and engage them in a dialogue on how to create a healthier culture, the process can be very encouraging and beneficial.

Next, create the plan. View the plan in a positive sense as an effort to enhance the health of firefighters. Avoid looking at the plan as a risk-reduction or punitive process.

Key points for developing an effective plan include the following:

- Define specific goals, objectives, and timelines for change.
- Evaluate where each firefighter currently stands. Determine not only where they are physically but also mentally. What is their attitude toward fitness and health? Are they willing to take the steps necessary to improve their health?

The Stages of Change model is a great tool to use.

- For each goal, designate a team of firefighters who will develop a plan for accomplishing the goal. Each group should have a fitness leader who will act as spokesperson for the group. Ideally, team leaders should have a passion for fitness and health.
- Avoid micromanaging: define the project or task, let the leader know the expectations, provide the necessary resources, offer feedback, then get out of the way and let your staff think through the process.
- Ensure that each team has a deadline for developing a plan. Plans will be presented at a general meeting, where all departmental members can hear and evaluate each plan.

Specific considerations for the plan should include the following:

- Does each shift allow for exercise time?
- Where will firefighters exercise? What types of equipment will be needed and where will the equipment be located (e.g., at every station or at acentral location)? Will a commercial health club or city fitness center be utilized?
- Are firefighters permitted to eat frequently (e.g., five to six times per day) or are they restricted to the traditional three meals per day?
- Who will be responsible for purchasing nutritious food, preparing meals, and so on?

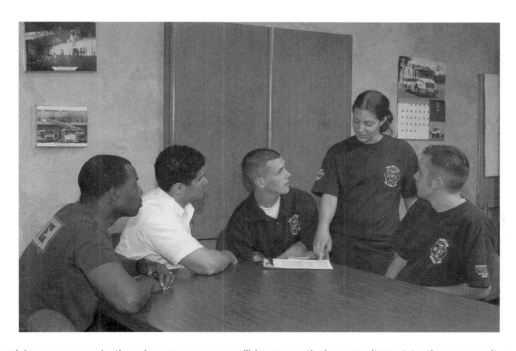

FIGURE 5-2   Involving everyone in the change process will increase their commitment to the new culture.

Step 4: Implement the Plan

This phase is about implementing the plans you have developed and providing people with the skills and support they need to be successful.

Fire chiefs must support the changes in ways beyond verbal support; they must lead the effort by changing their own behaviors if necessary. This will set the tone for the culture. Firefighters take their cues from their leaders, whether these cues are implicit or explicit. In addition, performance reviews should recognize healthy behaviors. If they are not recognized they will not be viewed as important.

Each firefighter has to make an individual decision to exercise and eat healthily. Provide reward ceremonies where individuals are recognized for improving their health status. Recognition should not be limited to highly successful individuals–every firefighter who makes an effort to improve his or her fitness and health levels should be recognized by peers.

Step 5: Evaluate Your Plan at Regular Intervals

Effective change is an ongoing cycle of exploration, understanding, and action. Review your plan regularly. Every three months conduct an analysis of how everyone is doing. Review every aspect of your plan. Every part of the plan must contribute to your overall goal. If it doesn't, modify or eliminate it.

Essentially, cultural change toward improved health means creating positive norms that produce healthy, innovative, and productive behaviors. You can change your department to a healthy department. Changing the culture requires time, commitment, planning, and proper execution–but it can be done. Clearly, individuals must assume responsibility for their own behavior and be held accountable. However, when firefighters know their department is actively helping them succeed in being healthy they will feel passionate, connected, and engaged in their work.

TOOLS AND TECHNIQUES FOR CULTURAL DEVELOPMENT

Developing healthy departmental cultures depends on generating ideas and helping individuals progressively improve their health levels. Following are three proven techniques that will help your planning groups become more effective.

- The Stages of Change Model
- Brainstorming
- Nominal Group Technique

The Stages of Change Model

An understanding of basic psychology will help firefighters change their unhealthy behaviors. The **Stages of Change model** demonstrates that individuals go through a specific order of changes before they are successful.[1] Originally developed to help people quit smoking, the Stages of Change model is now used to treat a host of behavioral problems, including overeating and physical inactivity.

The model has five stages that individuals go through before successfully changing their behavior:

- Precontemplation
- Contemplation
- Preparation
- Action
- Maintenance

Stage 1: Precontemplation

This is the stage at which individuals are not even considering a change in their behavior. Because they don't think they have a problem, precontemplators are not likely to seek help.

Strategy: Have a counselor or facilitator discuss the individual's health status. Cover the issues of healthy eating and weight loss. Discuss the topic but avoid getting into specific strategies. Stick to the facts—do not use opinions.

Stage 2: Contemplation

Individuals at this stage are thinking about making some change but may be somewhat ambivalent. They are more open to discussing adding healthy behaviors to their routine than are precontemplators.

Strategy: Create a decision balance sheet to identify the individual's motivating statements and potential barriers to change. Assess the individual's level of motivation and confidence. Start to build self-efficacy and teach the person how to problem solve.

Stage 3: Preparation

Preparation is the stage when people are on the verge of changing and have begun to investigate the options available to them. They are making the transition from thinking about doing healthy behaviors to actually doing healthy behaviors.

Strategy: Help the individual plan which changes to undertake. Set short-term goals based on motivating statements made on the decision balance sheet.

Stage 4: Action

The action stage starts when clients are ready to follow through with their goals.

Strategy: Provide positive reinforcement for any success. Get the individual to identify future goals. Suggest starting a food log or diary.

Stage 5: Maintenance

When the individual has followed through on their goals for at least six months they are considered to be at the maintenance level. Healthy behaviors have become second nature.

Strategy: Reinforce success and positive behavior. Explain the dangers of relapse and identify strategies for common situations that are likely to occur. Use coaching sessions to assist individuals in modifying old goals and creating new ones, as needed.

Brainstorming

The more brainpower you bring to bear on a problem, the smarter the solutions you're likely to get. Ideally, every group member would contribute both viable and non-workable ideas. However, in every group dominant personalities will intimidate some individuals from contributing. Here's a five step-plan for getting the most from your **brainstorming** sessions (**Figure 5-3**).

Step 1: Start with a goal that's clear and reachable. Make it clear that you're looking for as many ideas as possible. Alex Osborn, who coined the term "brainstorming," said that the most inspired concepts come from the most prolific groups.

Step 2: Keep the group small. Too big a group can get unwieldy and intimidating. Twelve should be the maximum number.

Step 3: Appoint a facilitator and notetaker. The facilitator is responsible for keeping the group moving along and on point. The notetaker should record ideas on a whiteboard so everyone can see what's been discussed. This allows the facilitator to return to an

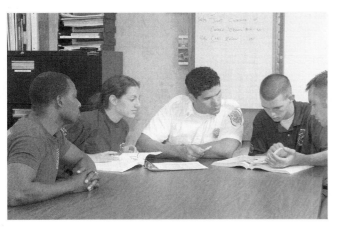

FIGURE 5-3 Generating ideas through brainstorming.

earlier thought and build on the most promising concepts. The facilitator is also responsible for generating participation from "wallflowers" by asking questions that play to their strengths. The facilitator might say, "You worked at a fitness center before. What can you tell us about equipment layout?"

Step 4: Think outside the box. This isn't always easy for departmental members so assemble a group that contains outsiders who have relevant experience in the area.

You might bring in a fitness professional for input on equipment purchases and biometric testing.

Step 5: Keep meetings short. Creativity tends to come in intense bursts, and meetings should last no longer than 60 minutes—or less.

Nominal Group Technique

Creativity won't flow unless people feel comfortable and not threatened when they offer up ideas. Reward risk, since risktakers are far more valuable to your department than those who play it safe. "It's impossible to come up with a few good ideas without generating a lot of bad ones," says Robert Sutton, professor of management at Stanford University. One method of maximizing each person's contribution is to use the **nominal group technique**.

1. Have every member write down their idea(s) on a sheet of paper.
2. Do not put names on the paper.
3. Put all the papers into a pile at the center of the table.
4. Each member draws a paper (not their own) from the pile.
5. Each member the reads the idea(s) listed on the paper.
6. The group evaluates the idea(s). Negative comments and remarks are not allowed.

The facilitator keeps the group on track by objectively evaluating the idea. Try to find the upside to every idea.

INDIVIDUAL CHANGE

Change is difficult. All of us who have tried to give up old habits and start new ones know how hard it is. Psychologists use the term **self-efficacy** in relation to behavior change. Self-efficacy is the amount of confidence an individual has in his or her own ability to carry out a desired behavior. You have a high level of self-efficacy if you feel confident in your ability to progress even amidst tempting situations. An effective way to develop self-efficacy and learn new behaviors is to use the S.M.A.R.T. goal-setting technique (see Chapter Two).

Determining What Stage You are In

The following question model will help you determine what stage of change you are in.

This model uses exercise as the question, but you could substitute nutrition, flossing, or any healthy behavior that is desired.

Stage	Behavior
Precontemplation	Does not exercise and does not plan to
Contemplation	Does not exercise but plans to sometime in the future
Preparation	Does not exercise but is planning to start in the next month
Action	Has exercised regularly for the past one to five months
Maintenance	Has exercised regularly for the past six months or more

Strategies for Moving Through the Stages of Change Model

Once you have determined what stage of change you are in, set goals by using the S.M.A.R.T. goal-setting technique. Post your goals in a prominent place (bulletin board, day planner, bathroom mirror, car dashboard, refrigerator, etc.) where you will see them every day.

Use the following strategies to help you progress through the stages:

Precontemplation, Contemplation, and Preparation

- Read and learn about the benefits of exercise
- Keep a daily time log to see when a workout could fit in
- Investigate how many calories are burned during exercise
- Map out a safe walking/cycling/running route
- Investigate exercise facilities
- Look at your high school pictures for inspiration
- Look at your latest blood profile
- List the pros and cons of daily exercise sessions
- List the benefits of losing weight

- Imagine what your health will be like in five years if you don't make any positive changes
- Publicly announce your intentions
- Create a plan of action
- Write and sign a behavioral change contract
- Keep a log, chart, or diary of your progress
- Post motivational signs, posters, and affirmations where you can see them daily.

Action and Maintenance

- Use positive self-talk
- Incorporate rewards for each goal accomplished
- Walk with your spouse rather than watching TV
- Practice relaxation rather than arguing or retaliating
- Drink water instead of soda
- Exercise instead of indulging in "happy hour"
- Have workout clothes ready and available
- Plan ahead by visualizing actions when confronted with a temptation
- Write a partner contract with goals and partner's commitments
- Work out with a partner
- Join a support group with others who are doing the same thing

---

PERFORMANCE POINT

What changes can you make in your own daily routine that will ultimately help make a positive change to your fire department's "fitness culture?" If it is your turn to prepare the dinner meal, what if you found a healthy and tasty recipe and provided it? Would others follow your lead? It is certainly possible. What if you asked your shift members to exercise with you? What if you made informal agreements with shift members about participating in an exercise plan or a weight-loss plan? Not only would the other members benefit, but others may eventually follow your lead as well.

In the case of fitness for firefighters, you do not have to be a victim of a poor fire department fitness culture. You can make a difference for yourself, and, possibly, be an instigator for cultural change on your shift, at your station, or even throughout the entire department.

EQUIPMENT SELECTION AND PURCHASE

Several factors need to be considered when selecting and purchasing exercise equipment:

Weight Machines

1. Cable systems should have plastic-coated cables, which are less likely to fray.
2. Movable attachments should not have soft metal pulleys.
3. Movable parts should be easily lubricated.
4. Frames should have the capacity to be anchored to the floor or wall.
5. Equipment should be coated with corrosion-resistant paint.
6. Safety stops in selectorized machines should be aligned.
7. Cotter pins should not be difficult to place in stacks.
8. Nonslip surfaces should surround lifting areas.
9. Lifting areas should be free of clutter.
10. Plates, bars, and collars should be stored after each use.
11. Preset barbells and dumbbells should be welded in place.
12. Free-standing benches should be sturdy enough to support anticipated loads and their bolts should be welded in place.
13. Bench surfaces should be padded to avoid splinters.
14. Safety stops for preventing injury should be designed into equipment.

Cardiovascular Equipment

1. Electrical plugs should be grounded. Ground fault interrupters should be on the power source.
2. Treadmills should have an emergency stop button on the handrail.
3. Countdown timers should automatically stop equipment.
4. Treadmills should have guardrails on three sides.
5. Instructions for safe use should be permanently mounted on units.
6. Preventive maintenance should be easily accomplished.
7. Touch heart rate sensors are only accurate at low intensities. The best way to track heart rate is to use a chest strap and receiver unit. Polar monitors are compatible with most cardiovascular training equipment.

Space Requirements

The amount of space available often determines the type or amount of equipment selected. When you consider the needs for space, you will need to take into account the circulation of participants and the average space needed for larger items like free weight racks, treadmills, single-station selectorized equipment, and smaller items like bikes. Most equipment manufacturers offer space-planning services that are invaluable, especially if you are planning on using only one brand of equipment.

A rule of thumb for designing exercise spaces is that one station or footprint of exercise equipment occupies approximately 46 square feet (4 square meters) of floor space.

Durability

There is no ironclad way to calculate the life expectancy of exercise equipment. The warranty on equipment serves as a rough indicator of its life expectancy. For example, manufacturers of selectorized strength equipment frequently warranty the structural frame for life, the moving parts for a year, and the upholstery for 90 days, because each material has a different projected life span.

From an accounting perspective, the usable life of most exercise equipment is about five years.

Cleaning and Maintenance

Once you have purchased the equipment, the endless process of cleaning and preventive maintenance begins.

Maintaining the equipment easily can add five years to a machine, maybe more. The usage patterns in a typical fire department are probably less than a commercial health club. However, if you have a couple of treadmills and they are always busy you will need to maintain them more often. The life span of equipment parts and materials can be short if proper maintenance procedures are not followed.

Set up a cleaning and preventive maintenance schedule. Electrical components and moisture are not well suited to one another. Take care to avoid sweating onto display boards and to secure bottle holders on equipment at a level well below any circuitry. Computerized display boards should only be cleaned with plain water and a clean rag. Commercial cleaning solutions may be used on all other surfaces. Consult with the manufacture if in doubt.

Guidelines for General Cleaning and Maintenance

Cardiovascular equipment

Daily cleaning:
Clean the electronic console with plain water and a clean cloth.

Weekly cleaning:
Clean the entire exterior with a disinfectant cleanser recommended by the equipment manufacturer.

Monthly cleaning:
Treadmills: Remove the cover and vacuum the motor electronic compartment.

Check the belt tension and tracking. Check the amperage draw as well to ensure that it is within the manufacturer's requirements. Raise the elevation and vacuum underneath.

Ellipticals: Remove the motor cover and vacuum the area surrounding the generator.

Stationary bikes: Remove the cover and vacuum the motor electronic compartment.

Quarterly cleaning:
Stepmills require quarterly cleaning and lubrication. Calling a specialist is recommended.

Resistance-training equipment
Daily/weekly:

Selectorized strength equipment: Wipe down the upholstery and inspect it for tears. Inspect the cable and handgrips for wear and clean the guide rods. Lubricate the guide rods with a Teflon spray. Never use WD-40 as a lubricant because it is a parts cleaner and will remove all the lubrication from the rods. Check the bolts, screws, and any hardware.

Plate-loaded strength equipment: Clean the upholstery and frame weekly. Check all hardware to ensure that all bolts and screws are tight.

Free weights: Clean upholstery on free-weight benches daily or weekly. Check the bolts, screws, and adjustment mechanisms on dumbbells, racks, and benches. Make sure that weight collars fit snugly and examine the weight plates for any cracks.

Cable machines: Cable must be checked for proper tension. If the cable is showing signs of cracks or fraying, replace it immediately. Failure to do this can cause damage to the nylon pulleys, or injury to users.

Cardiovascular Equipment Purchasing Guidelines

Treadmills. Treadmills are the bread-and-butter training machine for firefighters. You can walk, run, incline the unit, and perform many aerobic tests.

There are three categories of treadmills:

1. Club commercial: These treadmills are designed to handle the pounding and use of a variety of people. User weights can go up to 350 to 400 pounds. The treadmills can be run under a variety of conditions, and with proper care you probably won't need to ever purchase another unit. You will need an 110 volt, 20 amp dedicated outlet to run this kind of treadmill.

2. Standard commercial: These models give good durability and features but are not good choices for testing purposes. They are not as durable as the club commercial models, and eventually vibration and wear will take its toll on these models. User weights can go up to 300 pounds.

3. Light commercial: The downfall of these units are the lightweight frames and components, which aren't designed to handle vibration from numerous users of varying bodyweights and workout routines. User weights can go up to 225 to 250 pounds.

Treadmill specifications:

Look for units that have 4 horsepower with a speed range of 0.5 to 12 mph.

The unit should have elevation capability of 15 percent with 0.5 percent increments.

AC-drive treadmills are the best. Most of the best treadmills carry this type of motor platform and they are very reliable. DC-drive treadmills are also good and are found on standard-duty and light commercial treadmills. However, it is very expensive to replace the motor. For testing purposes, an AC drive will give you the most accurate speed control. On many treadmills 3 mph may be different depending on the weight of the person.

Look for a deck and belt that need no maintenance. Most commercial treadmills use maintenance-free systems. Stay away from treadmills that use waxing systems. The deck should run smoothly with minimal noise. It should be at least 20 inches wide, with 22 inches being better. A wider surface makes it safer for walking, running, and jogging. These wide platforms are more stable and the frames absorb energy better.

Deck suspension helps with absorbing energy. A spring-like suspension will cause your legs to fatigue when transferring workouts off the treadmill. An "orthopedic belt" is thicker; however, they don't last long and their ability to absorb energy is minimal.

The handrails should be sturdy and situated so that they do not interfere with user arm movements. Warranties on the motor, deck, rollers, and electronics should be at least two years; the frame warranty should be lifetime.

Incline Trainers. Incline trainers are an excellent choice for firefighters. The Free Motion Incline Trainer has all the features and workouts of a treadmill with one big advantage: you can incline this unit up to 30 percent to simulate hill or stair climbing. This unit is expensive, running about $5,300+ depending on which features are included. However, it is well worth the money.

Stationary Bikes. Bikes fall into two categories: Club commercial and light commercial. Club commercial bikes have a more comfortable fit for all sized riders, they offer a wide variety of programs, and the components underneath the shroud are heavier and of better quality. You will also have a greater resistance range with a club commercial product, along with a bearing and crankshaft designed to handle bigger, stronger riders whose workouts demand this quality. Commercial bikes carry more inertia within their drive system, giving you a smooth and consistent ride, especially when working out in the high resistance range. Another plus is that most bikes produced today run cordless.

Heart rate measurement capability is recommended for testing and training programs.

Spin bikes are a great option in the upright bike category. They have a great resistance range and are durable. They have no programs, but the newer models have an optional computer that measures rpm, heart rate, distance, and time. A quality bike will cost from $1,500 to $2,500.

Elliptical Trainers. An elliptical trainer is usually the third choice for a fire department. Many have optional arm movement handles. Look for units that have a smooth motion; some have a flat spot at the top of the movement that makes it feel jerky. A good way to feel the motion of the ellipse is to see if it's as smooth going backward as going forward. Standard commercial models run $2,500 on up.

Stepmill. This is the ultimate workout machine for firefighters. It is unlike most stairclimbers in that users move their bodyweight in an upward motion. A big plus is that it has the CPAT and NYFD test protocols built in. Stepmills are expensive, running about $4,500. However, they are well worth the expense.

Recommendations for Functional Training and Testing Equipment Purchases

- Fit Ball: choose burst-resistant types. The size of the Fit Ball is determined by the height of the individual, **Figure 5-4**.
- Vertical jump height: Vertec is the most popular device for testing vertical jump height.
- Body composition testing: Lange skinfold calipers are the most popular. Cheap calipers are not recommended. Bioelectric Impedance systems (scale,

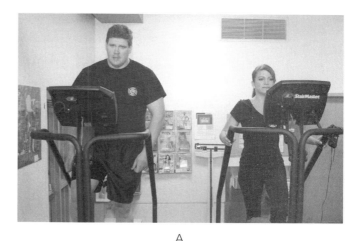

A

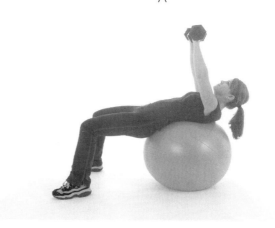

B

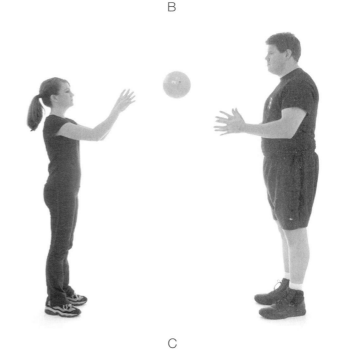

C

FIGURE 5-4 Fit balls and medicine balls provide great workout options.

handheld devices) are not recommended because they are not accurate for lean and athletic populations.

CASE STUDIES

The West Metro Fire Department

In 1999, the West Metro Fire Protection District, located in the western part of the Denver metropolitan area, found that 43 of its 240 firefighters measured as clinically obese and 9 were morbidly obese. Additionally, 25 percent of the firefighters couldn't meet the minimum aerobic standard. "A lot of people were overweight, were on medications, were meeting with doctors on a regular basis," said Bob Stratman, Wellness Director.

Cpt. Jim Thatcher, 53, was a prime example. "If I had the choice between exercise or TV, it was always TV," he said. "I was always tired. I got exhausted pretty easily and I would find easier ways to do something instead of the right way." His love of food and lack of exercise pushed his 5-foot 8-inch frame to 286 pounds.

In 2006, 5-foot, 8-inch Eric Bates weighed 205 pounds. "If I got hungry I'd go to Good Times Hamburgers. It was hard to get motivated. It was a workout just to get to the workout." When they ate together, the firefighters had no concept of what was involved in healthy nutrition. "We'd eat pasta, bread, and dessert," Lt. Dustin Horn said.

In 1999, Stratman and a task force of firefighters developed a plan to change the exercise and nutritional habits of the department. Working with the University of Colorado's physiology and nutrition lab, they interviewed the firefighters on their fitness and food habits. They also used heart rate monitors to track the firefighter's energy expenditure (calories burnt) when performing firefighter tasks such as raising a ladder and climbing stairs. For example, a 180-pound man fighting a fire for 12 minutes burns approximately 420 calories. From this data they developed exercises that would not only help firefighters lose weight but also increase their conditioning for firefighting duties.

Highlights of the plan include the following:

- Through a government grant, West Metro put exercise equipment in all of its stations. A full gym was updated at headquarters and is available to all departmental personnel.

- A core-strengthening video was developed and copies were put in all stations
- Firefighters use the software program Fitday to track their meals and exercise participation.
- Cookbooks were developed with comparisons of healthy recipes and fast food offerings.

The efforts are paying off. Since the change began, the district has seen a reduction in body fat and an increase in core strengthening and aerobic capacity. Some of the results are shown below:

Test/year	1999	2007
Clinically obese	43	6
Aerobic standard	72 failed	0 failed
Workers compensation claims	200–300	35

Firefighters now focus on making healthy meals, with dishes such as chicken club sandwiches, salad, and fruit. "A typical morning is egg whites, fresh fruit, and a little bacon for protein," Stratman says—a major improvement from a menu that typically had included a lot of bacon, butter, biscuits, and gravy.

Thatcher lost 30 pounds by following the plan. "It's easier to breathe. My knees don't hurt as much. I feel good. I want to lose another 30 pounds," he said. Bates lost 18 pounds and lowered his body fat by 5.65 percent.

West Metro was recently honored with the 2007 Fire Service Organizational Safety Award by the International Association of Fire Chiefs, given annually to acknowledge a department's health, fitness, and safety.

Case study question: What steps of the cultural change process did the West Metro Fire District follow when changing their culture?

- Flexibility tester: The Accuflex I measures both the standard test and the modified test that allows for limb length.
- Biofoam rollers: used for massage and alignment.
- BOSU: recommended for training balance and core stability.

- Medicine balls: essentially weighted balls of various types. They range in weight from 2-30 pounds (see **Figure 5-4**).
- Disc pillows: strengthen the muscles that stabilize ankles, knees, core, and shoulders.

CHAPTER SUMMARY

A fire department's culture has a dramatic influence on the fitness and health of its firefighters. A culture that promotes health, innovation, and productivity will enable firefighters to take active roles in improving their health. A five-step process enables fire chiefs to evaluate how their present culture affects the health of firefighters and how to develop strategies that increase individual and departmental health efforts. First, a vision of what an ideal culture looks like is developed. Next, the present culture is evaluated and plans are developed to create the ideal culture. Finally, when implementing the plan, it is important to get every firefighter involved in this process by assigning them specific tasks that are designed to move the department toward the ideal culture. Each firefighter must be trained in the skills and given the support they need to be successful. Two effective methods of getting firefighters involved are brainstorming and the nominal group technique. Both methods focus on generating ideas in a non-intimidating manner by emphasizing contribution and minimizing criticism. The final step is to evaluate the plan at regular intervals.

It is important to identify each firefighter's level of self-efficacy—the amount of confidence an individual has in his or her own ability to carry out a desired behavior. Firefighters with higher self-efficacy levels will be more successful in developing and maintaining healthy behaviors. An effective technique is to use the Stages of Change model that outlines the stages or phases that individuals go through when successfully changing their behavior. Once it is determined what stage of change an individual is in (precontemplation, contemplation, preparation, action, or maintenance), strategies are formulated to help the individual move to the next stage. An integral part of this process is to set goals using the S.M.A.R.T. goal-setting technique.

Several factors need to be considered when selecting and purchasing exercise equipment, including safety, space requirements, durability, cleaning and maintenance.

Treadmills and stepmills are ideally suited for training firefighters. Most individuals are able to walk or run at varying inclines, and treadmills have many aerobic performance tests built into their programs. The Stairmaster Step Mill has both the NYFD aerobic capacity test and the CPAT firefighter candidate-testing protocol.

KEY TERMS

Brainstorming An idea-generating group session

Culture Beliefs and standards that govern behavior in an organization

Nominal group technique Method of maximizing each member's contribution to group idea generation

Self-efficacy The amount of confidence an individual has in their ability to carry out a desired behavior

Stages of change model Process that an individual goes through when changing their behavior

CHECK YOUR LEARNING

1. The most important consideration when purchasing exercise equipment is
   a. safety.
   b. space requirements.
   c. durability.
   d. ease of cleaning.

2. Fitness and health levels of firefighters depend on
   a. their decisions to eat and exercise healthfully.
   b. the support of their peers.
   c. support from the fire chief.
   d. availability of exercise equipment.
   e. all of the above.

3. The first step in developing a cultural change plan is to
   a. evaluate where the department is at now.
   b. develop the plan.
   c. envision what the department should look like.
   d. recruit support personnel.

4. The developmental team is formed during what cultural change step?
   a. step 1
   b. step 2
   c. step 3
   d. step 4
   e. step 5

5. An individual who is thinking about changing their behavior is in what stage?
   a. precontemplation
   b. contemplation
   c. preparation
   d. action
   e. maintenance

6. Which type of cardiovascular equipment is considered the "bread and butter" training mode for firefighters?
   a. bike
   b. incline trainer
   c. stepmill
   d. elliptical trainer
   e. treadmill

7. What type of treadmill is recommended for firefighters?
   a. light commercial
   b. club commercial
   c. standard commercial
   d. industrial commercial

8. In what stage of change is an individual whose exercise and healthy eating have become habits?
   a. precontemplation
   b. contemplation
   c. preparation
   d. action
   e. maintenance

9. Performance reviews and individual recognition ceremonies are conducted during which step(s) of the cultural change process?
   a. step 1
   b. step 2
   c. step 3
   d. steps 1 and 3
   e. steps 4 and 5

10. Developing a cultural change plan involves
   a. setting specific goals
   b. involving the entire staff
   c. evaluating each firefighter's physical condition
   d. assigning a team of firefighters to develop and accomplish each goal
   e. all of the above

REFERENCE

1. Prochaska, J.O., DiClemente, C.C., and Norcross, J.C. "In search of how people change: Applications to addictive behaviors." *American Psychologist* 47 (1992): 1102–11.

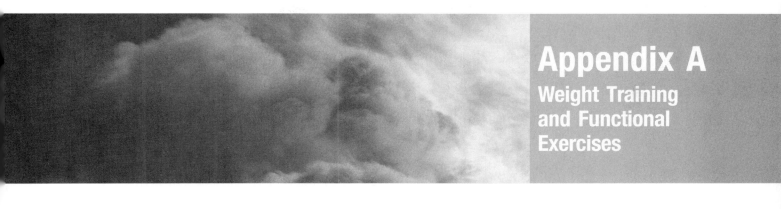

CHEST EXERCISES

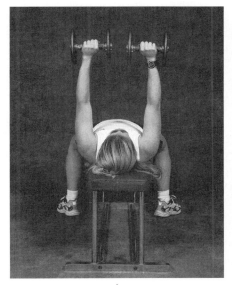 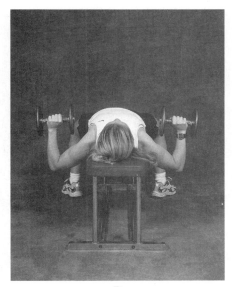

A   B

FIGURE A-1 Dumbbell press

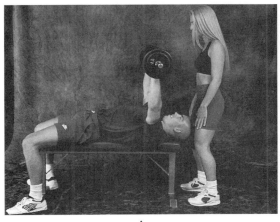 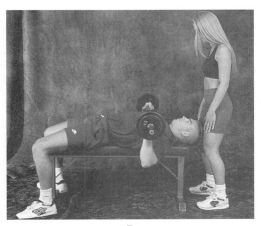

A   B

FIGURE A-2 Barbell press

CHEST EXERCISES

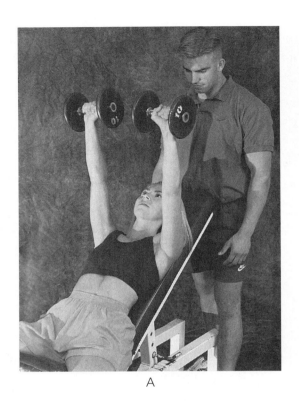
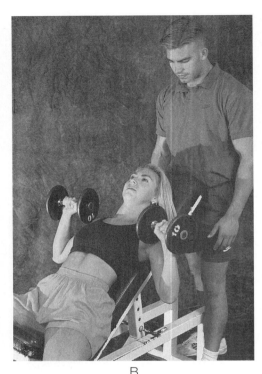

A   B

FIGURE A-3   Incline dumbbell press

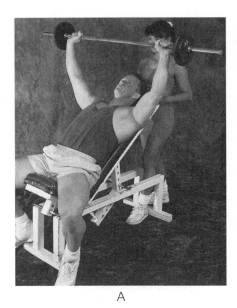
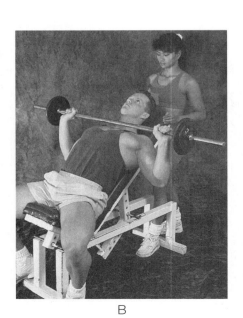

A   B

FIGURE A-4   Incline barbell press

BACK EXERCISES

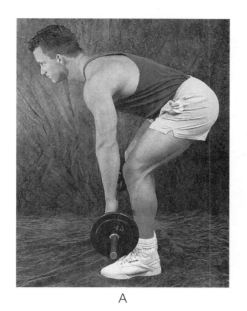 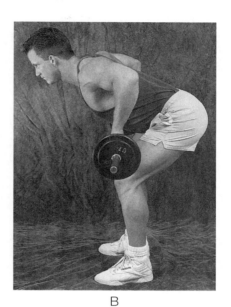

A   B

FIGURE A-5   Barbell bent over row

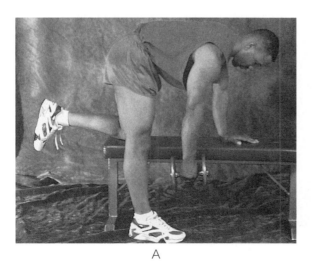 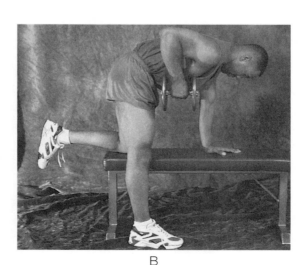

A   B

FIGURE A-6   One-dumbbell bent over row

BACK EXERCISES

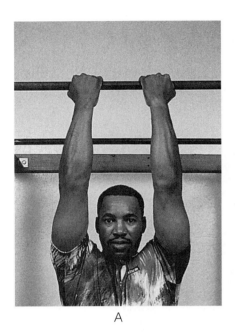 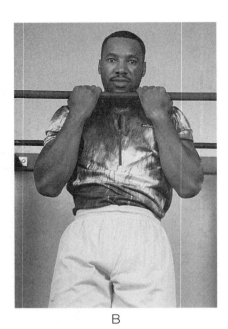

A   B

FIGURE A-7   Reverse grip chin-up

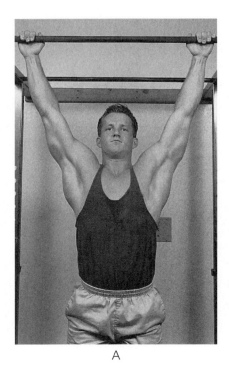 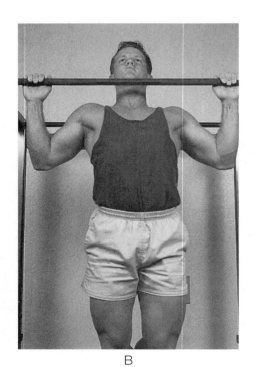

A   B

FIGURE A-8   Forward grip pull-up

BACK AND SHOULDER EXERCISES

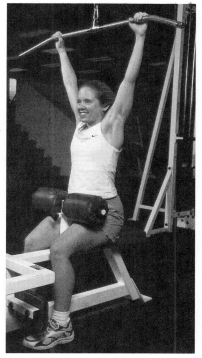
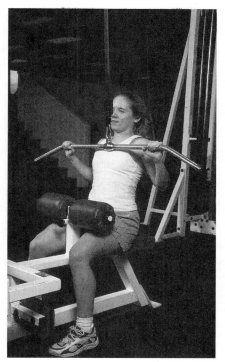

A   B

FIGURE A-9 Lat pull downs

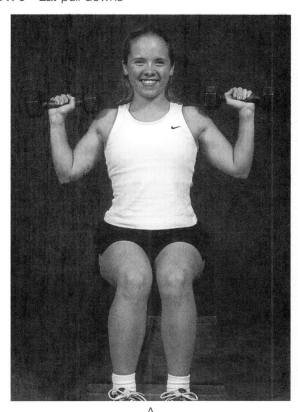
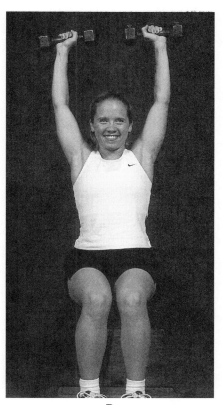

A   B

FIGURE A-10 Dumbbell overhead press

SHOULDER AND BICEP EXERCISES

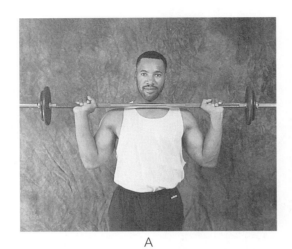

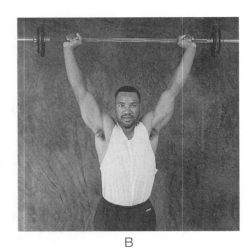

A   B

FIGURE A-11   Barbell overhead press

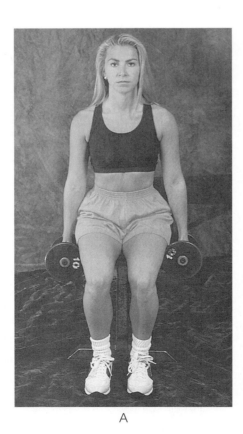

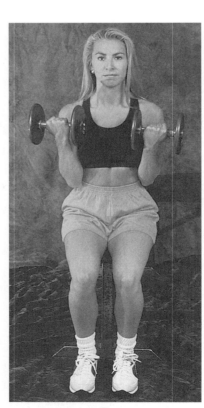

A   B

FIGURE A-12   Seated dumbbell curl

BICEP AND FOREARM EXERCISES

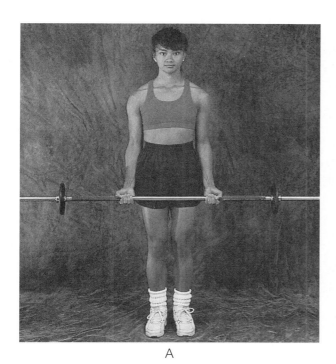
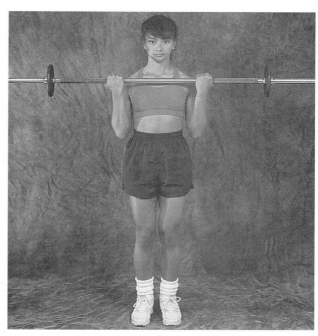

A   B

FIGURE A-13   Barbell curl

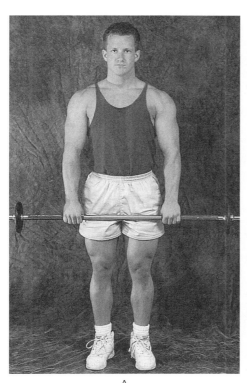
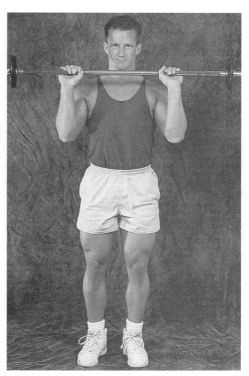

A   B

FIGURE A-14   Reverse curl

BICEP AND TRICEP EXERCISES

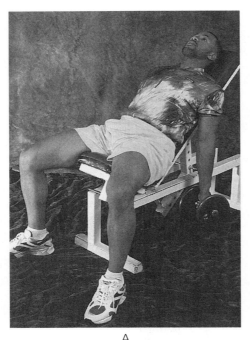 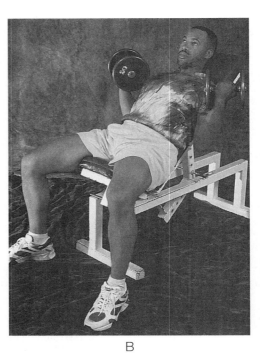

A   B

FIGURE A-15 Incline dumbbell curl

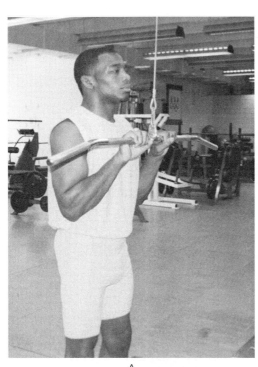 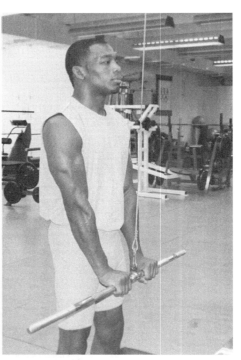

A   B

FIGURE A-16 Tricep pushdowns

TRICEP EXERCISES

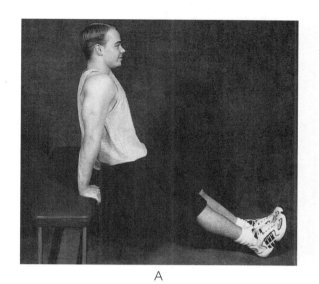
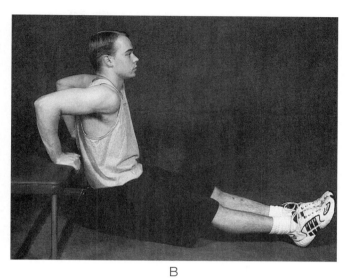

A   B

FIGURE A-17   Bench dips

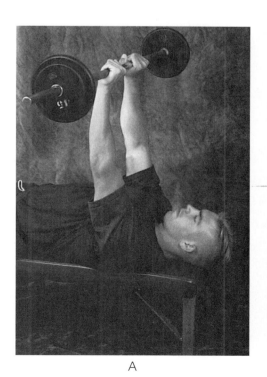
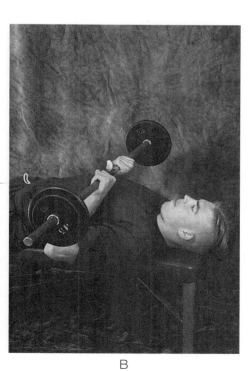

A   B

FIGURE A-18   Close grip bench press

LEG AND BACK EXERCISES

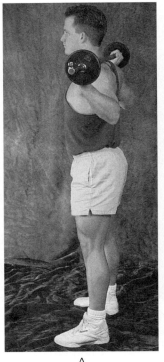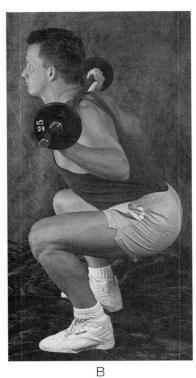

A   B

FIGURE A-19 Barbell squat

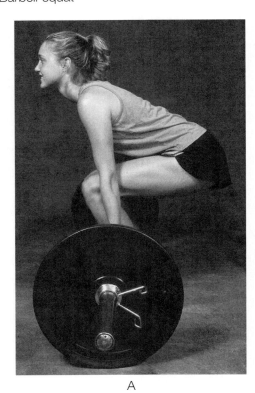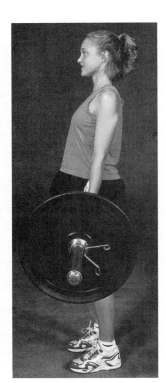

A   B

FIGURE A-20 Deadlift

LEG EXERCISES

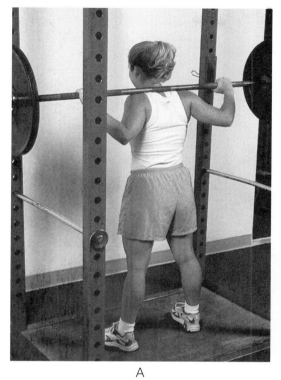 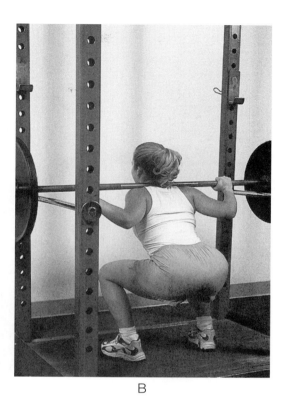

A	B

FIGURE A-21 Barbell squat

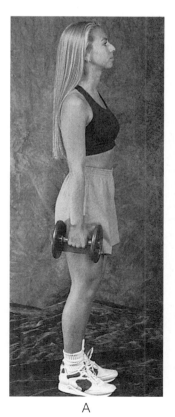 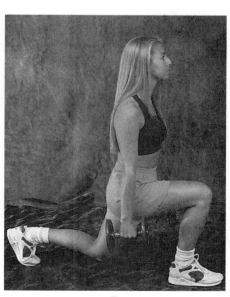

A	B

FIGURE A-22 Lunge

LEG EXERCISES

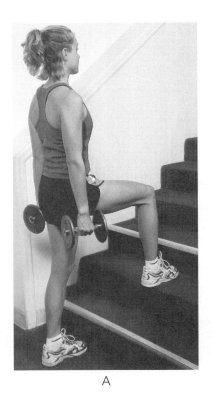
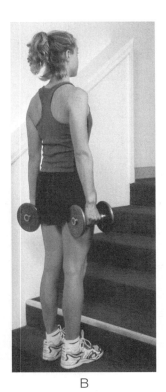

A   B

FIGURE A-23   Step up with dumbbells

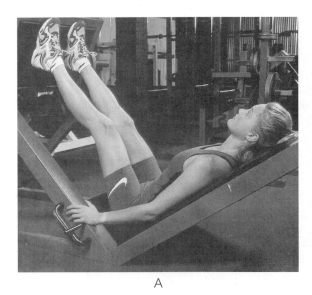
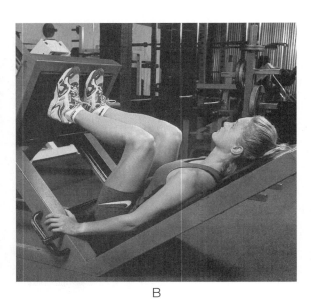

A   B

FIGURE A-24   Leg press

LEG EXERCISES

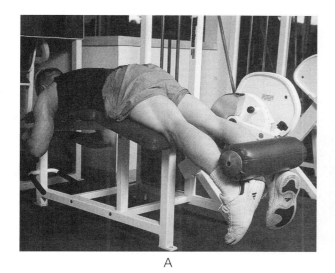
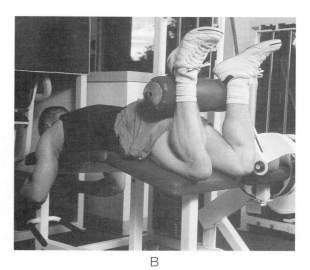

A

B

FIGURE A-25 Leg curl

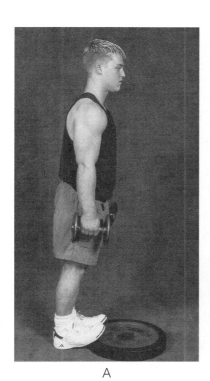
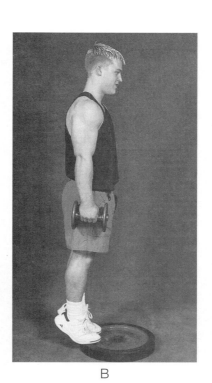

A

B

FIGURE A-26 Dumbbell calf raise

ABDOMINAL EXERCISES

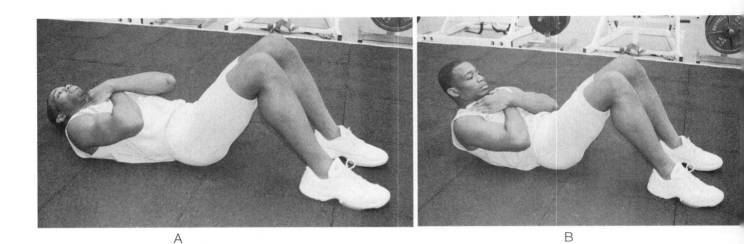

A   B

FIGURE A-27   Crunches

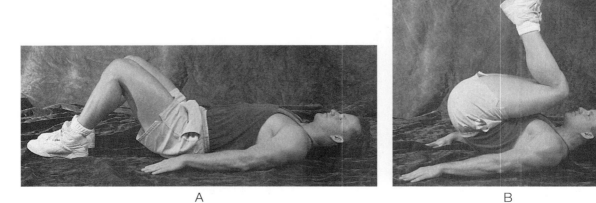

A   B

FIGURE A-28   Reverse crunches

ABDOMINAL EXERCISES

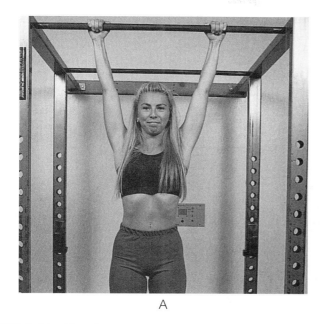
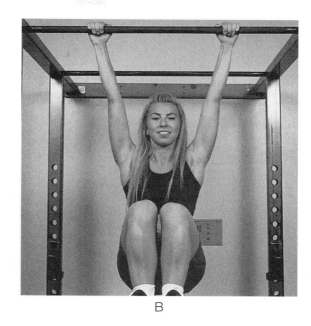

A

B

FIGURE A-29   Hanging knee raises

FUNCTIONAL EXERCISES

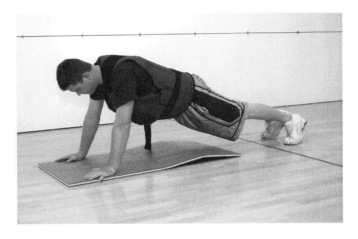

FIGURE B-1 Plank

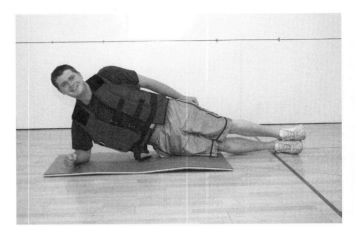

FIGURE B-2 Side plank

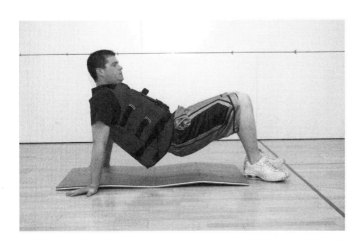

FIGURE B-3 Reverse plank

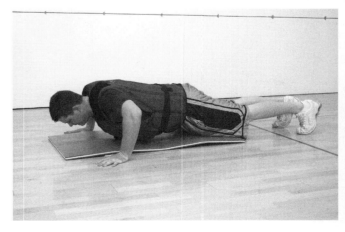

FIGURE B-4 Push-up

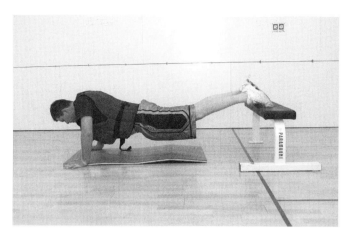

FIGURE B-5   Incline push-up

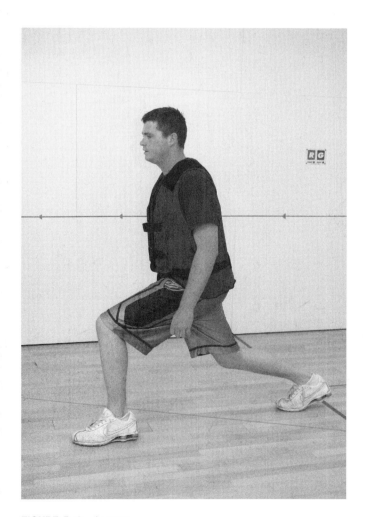

FIGURE B-6   Lunge

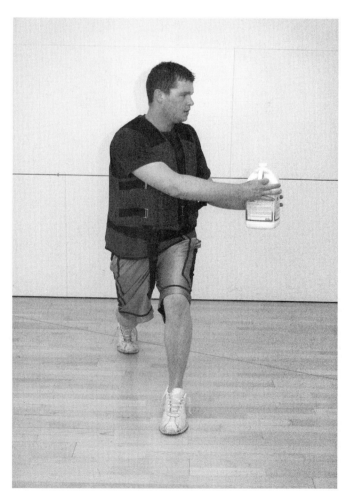

FIGURE B-7   Lunge with rotation

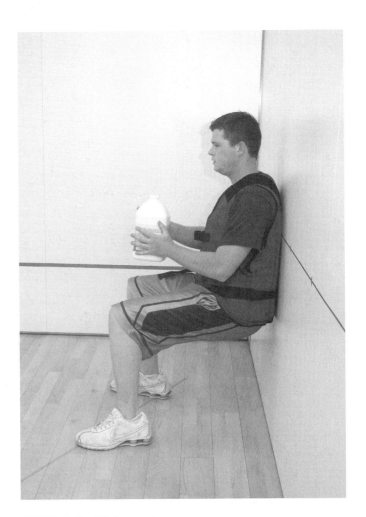

FIGURE B-8   Wall squat

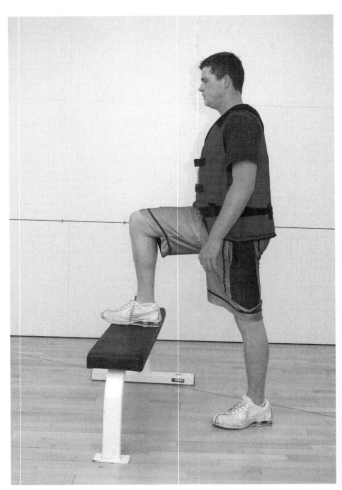

FIGURE B-9   Bench step-up—start

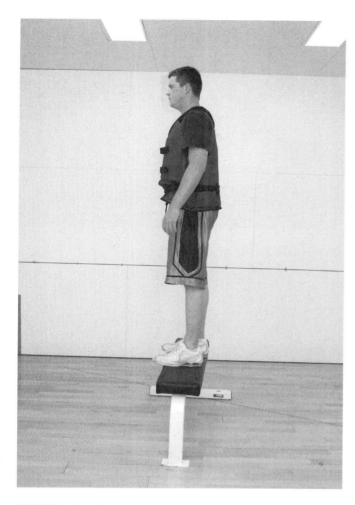

FIGURE B-10 Bench step-up—end

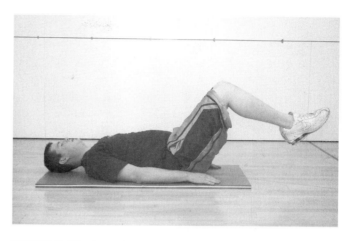

FIGURE B-12 Leg drop

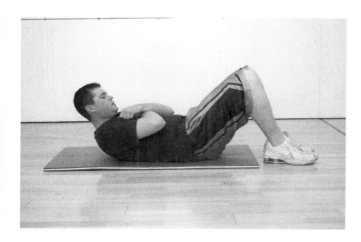

FIGURE B-11 Crunch

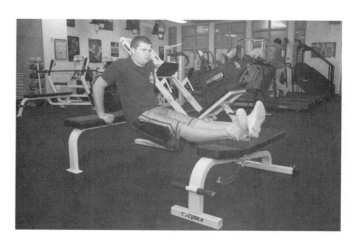

FIGURE B-13 Bench dips

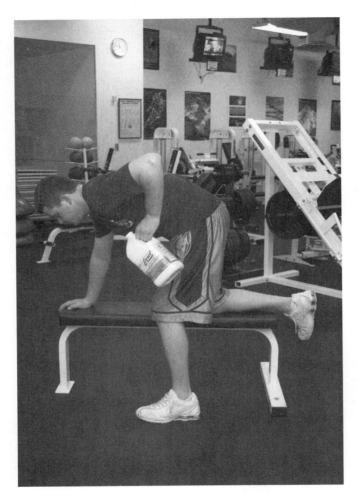

FIGURE B-14   Rowing

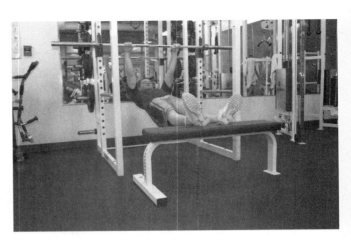

FIGURE B-16   Inverted row—ending position

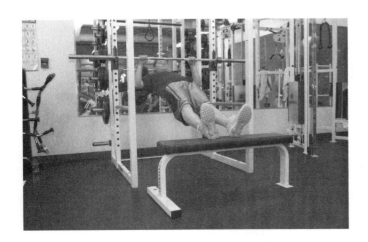

FIGURE B-15   Inverted row—top position

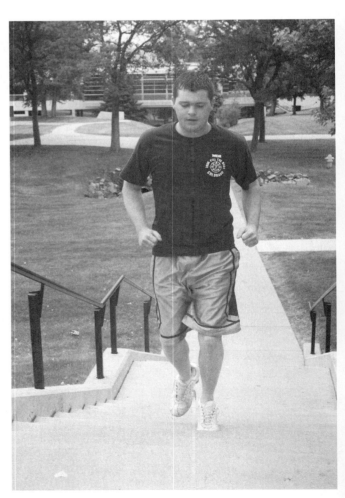

FIGURE B-17   Stair running

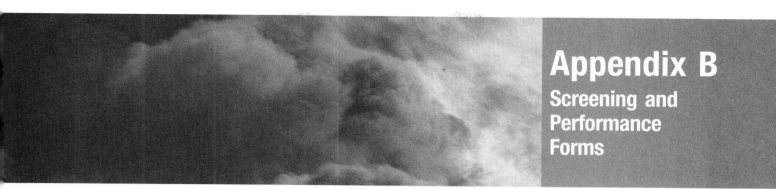

HEALTH SCREENING

1. Coronary Artery Disease Risk Factors

			Test Dates		
Cholesterol	Acceptable level	Ideal level	Test 1	Test 2	Test 3
Total Cholesterol	<200	<160	_____	_____	_____
HDL Cholesterol	>45	>60	_____	_____	_____
LDL Cholesterol	<100	<60	_____	_____	_____
Coronary Risk Ratio	<3.5	<3.0	_____	_____	_____
Triglycerides	<150	<90	_____	_____	_____
Blood Glucose	<90	<70	_____	_____	_____
Smoking	non-smoker		_____	_____	_____
Blood Pressure	systolic	diastolic	Test 1	Test 2	Test 3
Ideal	<110	<70	_____	_____	_____
Average	<120	<80			
Pre-Hypertension	121–39	81–89			
Stage 1 Hypertension	140–59	90–99			
Stage 2 Hpertension	160+	100+			
Height			_____	_____	_____
Body weight			_____	_____	_____
Body Mass Index (BMI)			_____	_____	_____
Body Composition Male:	<20%	<15%	_____	_____	_____
Body Composition Female:	<24%	<20%	_____	_____	_____

2. Medical Factors

_____ Rheumatic fever	_____ Heart murmur	_____ Chest pain
_____ Heart attack	_____ Leg pain	_____ Ulcers
_____ Emphysema	_____ Bronchitis	_____ Asthma
_____ Irregular heartbeat	_____ Thyroid	_____ Colitis
_____ Swollen ankles/calves	_____ Seizures	_____ Fainting
_____ Diabetes Type 2/Type 1		

3. Orthopedic

Condition	Effect on exercise and firefighter performance
Back injury	_____
Knee injury	_____
_____	_____
_____	_____

4. Medications

Medication	Effect on exercise and firefighter performance
_____	_____
_____	_____
_____	_____
_____	_____

5. Family History

_____ Heart attack	_____ Diabetes Type 2/ Type 1
_____ Obesity	_____ High blood pressure

BIOMETRIC TESTING

Test	Standard M: male F: female	Baseline date:	Retest 1 date:	Retest 2 date:	Retest 3 date:
Resting heart rate	<60	_____	_____	_____	_____
Body composition	M<15 F<20	_____	_____	_____	_____
Body mass index	<25	_____	_____	_____	_____
Waist-to-hip ratio	M<.95 F<.81	_____	_____	_____	_____
Balance	pass all tests	_____	_____	_____	_____
Pull-ups	M>10 F>5	_____	_____	_____	_____
Inverted row	M>10 F>4	_____	_____	_____	_____
Vertical jump	M>20 F>15	_____	_____	_____	_____
Leg press	M>1.7 F>1.5	_____	_____	_____	_____
Stepmill FDNY	M>42 F>38	_____	_____	_____	_____
Treadmill sub-max	M>5:00	_____	_____	_____	_____
Treadmill sub-max	F>5:00	_____	_____	_____	_____
Bench press 1RM	M>1 F>.7	_____	_____	_____	_____
Hand-grip strength	M>45 F>30	_____	_____	_____	_____
Push-ups					
Age 18–35	M: 42 F: 20	_____	_____	_____	_____
Age 36–52	M: 36 F: 15	_____	_____	_____	_____
Age 53+	M: 29 F: 11	_____	_____	_____	_____
Curl-ups					
Age 18–34	M: 70 F: 70	_____	_____	_____	_____
Age 35–50	M: 50 F: 50	_____	_____	_____	_____
Age 51+	M: 36 F: 36	_____	_____	_____	_____
Flexibility					
Age 20–29	M: 16 F: 18	_____	_____	_____	_____
Age 30–39	M: 15 F: 16.5	_____	_____	_____	_____
Age 40–49	M: 14.5 F: 16	_____	_____	_____	_____
Age 50+	M: 14 F:15	_____	_____	_____	_____

NUTRITION

1. Daily energy requirements

Use the chart below to determine your recommended number of daily calories needed. This chart is based upon an active firefighter who exercises 5–6 times per week.

Age	Male	Female
20–29	body weight x 23	body weight x 21
30–39	body weight x 22	body weight x 21
40–49	body weight x 22	body weight x 20
50–59	body weight x 21	body weight x 20
60+	body weight x 20	body weight x 19

Your body weight _____ × factor_____ = _____ Total daily calories needed

2. Determine how many calories are needed from each nutrient category

Total daily calories needed	_____
65% from carbohydrate	_____
20% from protein	_____
15% from fat	_____

3. Nutrient checklist

	Servings per day	Mon	Tue	Wed	Thr	Fri	Sat	Sun
whole grains	8–10	____	____	____	____	____	____	____
fruits	4	____	____	____	____	____	____	____
vegetables	5	____	____	____	____	____	____	____
water	8+	____	____	____	____	____	____	____
good fats	2	____	____	____	____	____	____	____
nuts	2	____	____	____	____	____	____	____
protein	4	____	____	____	____	____	____	____

MENTAL TRAINING

Use this chart to develop a mental-training strategy for your exercise sessions and firefighter duties.

Check

_____ Have you set goals for each practice session?

_____ Did your preparation help you to meet your goals?

_____ Do you visualize yourself executing each exercise session with perfect technique?

_____ Are you using positive self-talk?

_____ Do you perform relaxation techniques daily?

_____ Do you have a focus point for each exercise?

_____ Can you maintain your best focus when faced with distractions?

_____ Do you seek out and accept the feedback from your instructors, coaches, and fellow firefighters?

_____ Do you control any negative emotions?

_____ Do you have the discipline to follow your training schedule?

_____ Do you have a support system developed?

_____ Do you train with a "relaxed focus" and allow your body to execute the skills you have trained it to do?

_____ Do you sustain your focus through each workout?

_____ Do you center yourself before performing each exercise?

_____ Are you using "trigger" words to start the centering process?

CHECKLIST OF HEALTHY BEHAVIORS

_____ execute an exercise plan

_____ eat breakfast every day

_____ eat 5–6 meals per day

_____ eat a post-exercise meal of protein and carbohydrates

_____ floss teeth daily and see a dentist regularly

_____ get 10–20 minutes of sun daily

_____ take all necessary medicines and take them correctly in relation to food

_____ read food labels

_____ do not take unnecessary vitamins and supplements

_____ avoid exposure to passive smoke

_____ eliminate or minimize saturated fat

_____ eliminate trans fats

_____ drink alcohol in moderation

_____ take a multivitamin daily

_____ take a calcium and vitamin D supplement daily

_____ eat tomato paste and sauce 2–3 times weekly

GOAL SETTING

Set your goals below using the SMART goal-setting technique.

Goal 1

Specific	What exactly is to be done?	_____
Measurable	How will you evaluate progress?	_____
Attainable	Is the goal realistic?	_____
Relevant	Why is this goal important?	_____
Time-bound	What is the completion date?	_____

Objectives   Completion date

1. _____   _____

2. _____   _____

3. _____   _____

Feedback source _____

Goal 2

Specific	What exactly is to be done?	_____
Measurable	How will you evaluate progress?	_____
Attainable	Is the goal realistic?	_____
Relevant	Why is this goal important?	_____
Time-bound	What is the completion date?	_____

Objectives   Completion date

1. _____   _____

2. _____   _____

3. _____   _____

Feedback source _____

Goal 3

Specific	What exactly is to be done?	_____
Measurable	How will you evaluate progress?	_____
Attainable	Is the goal realistic?	_____
Relevant	Why is this goal important?	_____
Time-bound	What is the completion date?	_____

Objectives   Completion date

1. _____   _____

2. _____   _____

3. _____   _____

Feedback source _____

TRAINING SCHEDULE

Training phase: _____   Starting date: _____   Ending date: _____

Warmup	Mon	Tue	Wed	Thur	Fri	Sat	Sun
Mode/time	_____	_____	_____	_____	_____	_____	_____

Cardiovascular	Mon	Tue	Wed	Thur	Fri	Sat	Sun
Mode	_____	_____	_____	_____	_____	_____	_____
Time	_____	_____	_____	_____	_____	_____	_____
Intensity level	_____	_____	_____	_____	_____	_____	_____

Resistance training   Weight used/sets/reps

Exercises	Mon	Tue	Wed	Thur	Fri	Sat	Sun
_____	_____	_____	_____	_____	_____	_____	_____
_____	_____	_____	_____	_____	_____	_____	_____
_____	_____	_____	_____	_____	_____	_____	_____
_____	_____	_____	_____	_____	_____	_____	_____
_____	_____	_____	_____	_____	_____	_____	_____
_____	_____	_____	_____	_____	_____	_____	_____
_____	_____	_____	_____	_____	_____	_____	_____
_____	_____	_____	_____	_____	_____	_____	_____

Functional training   Sets/reps

Exercises	Mon	Tue	Wed	Thr	Fri	Sat	Sun
_____	_____	_____	_____	_____	_____	_____	_____
_____	_____	_____	_____	_____	_____	_____	_____
_____	_____	_____	_____	_____	_____	_____	_____
_____	_____	_____	_____	_____	_____	_____	_____

Flexibility

Stretches performed	Mon	Tue	Wed	Thr	Fri	Sat	Sun
_____	_____	_____	_____	_____	_____	_____	_____
_____	_____	_____	_____	_____	_____	_____	_____
_____	_____	_____	_____	_____	_____	_____	_____

CULTURAL DEVELOPMENT WORKSHEET

Step 1: What is your ideal work culture?

1. List ideas generated from meetings and surveys of the department   _____

2. Points to consider:

What types of exercise equipment are needed?   _____

Who will buy and maintain the equipment?   _____

Who will train employees?   _____

Will testing and counseling be provided for employees?   _____

Step 2: Where do you stand now?

1. Using data from meetings and surveys, assess firefighter's perceptions of the current departmental culture and how it affects fitness and health.

_____

_____

_____

_____

Step 3: Plan out the change

1. Share the results of the first two steps with the department.   _____

2. Get everyone involved in planning how to achieve a new culture.   _____

3. Set specific goals and timelines for each step.   _____

4. Assign each goal to a group.   _____

5. Provide training for your group leaders.   _____

Step 4: Implement the changes

1. Leaders must model new cultural standards.   _____

2. Recognize and reward firefighter's efforts toward exhibiting healthy behaviors.   _____

3. Reinforce new standards with training sessions, discussions, and support from all departmental staff.   _____

Step 5: Evaluate your new culture

1. Evaluate the departmental culture constantly. Conduct surveys on the effectiveness of your efforts toward change. Are your goals being realized?

_____

_____

_____

_____

_____

Appendix C
Equipment Specifications and Maintenance

EQUIPMENT SELECTION AND LAYOUT

Weight Machines and Training Area

_____ There should be floor space of approximately 46 square feet (4 square meters) for each piece of equipment

_____ There should be easy access to each piece of equipment of at least 36 inches between machines to accommodate lightweight wheelchairs

_____ Warranty on structural frame for life, the moving parts for a year, and the upholstery for 90 days should be available for each applicable piece of equipment

_____ Cable systems should have plastic-coated cables, which are less likely to fray

_____ There should be double stitching on padding. No staples should be used

_____ Movable attachments should not have soft metal pulleys

_____ Movable parts should be easily lubricated

_____ Movable parts should be enclosed to reduce cleaning and maintenance

_____ Frames should have the capacity to be anchored to the floor or wall

_____ Equipment should be coated with corrosion-resistant paint

_____ Safety stops in selectorized machines should be aligned

_____ Cotter pins should not be difficult to place in stacks

_____ Nonslip surfaces should surround lifting areas

_____ Lifting areas should be free of clutter

_____ Adequate storage for plates, bars, and collars

_____ Preset barbells and dumbbells should be welded in place

_____ Free-standing benches should be sturdy enough to support anticipated loads and their bolts should be welded in place

_____ Bench surfaces should be padded to avoid splinters

_____ Safety stops for preventing injury should be designed into equipment

_____ Power racks and cable crossovers should be secured to floor and wall

Cardiovascular Equipment and Layout

_____ Floor space of approximately 46 square feet (4 square meters) for each piece of equipment is needed

_____ Easy access to each piece of equipment of 36 inches to accommodate lightweight wheelchairs

_____ Electrical plugs should be grounded

_____ Treadmills should have an emergency stop button on the handrail

_____ Countdown timers should automatically stop equipment

_____ Treadmills should have guardrails on three sides

_____ Elliptical trainers should have a smooth motion

_____ Instructions for their safe use should be permanently mounted on all units

_____ Preventive maintenance should be easily accomplished

_____ Polar heart rate monitor compatible

Cardiovascular purchasing guidelines

Treadmills

_____ 110 volt 20 amp dedicated outlet

_____ Should accommodate user weights up to at least 300lbs. Standard commercial recommended

_____ 4 horsepower with a speed range of 0.5 to 12 mph

_____ Elevation capability of 15% with 0.5% increments

_____ AC-drive treadmills are the best

_____ Maintenance-free deck and belt

_____ Belt should run smoothly with minimal noise

_____ Deck should be at least 20" wide, with 22" recommended

_____ Handrails sturdy and do not interfere with arm movements

_____ Warranties on all components should be at least two years with a lifetime warranty on the frame

Other cardiovascular equipment:

_____ Before purchase, perform "test run" on stationary bikes, elliptical trainers, stairclimbers, and so on

_____ Upright and recumbent bikes should be cordless (electricity not required) and be capable of measuring heart rate by hand grip or heart rate monitor with chest strap

_____ Stepmill should have CPAT and NYFD test protocols built in. It is cost prohibitive to have these features installed

Functional training and testing equipment

_____ Fit Ball, burst-resistant, in varying sizes

_____ Vertec vertical jump tester

_____ Body composition testing—Lange skinfold calipers

_____ Flexibility tester—The Accuflex

_____ Biofoam rollers

_____ BOSU balance and stability trainer

_____ Medicine balls of varying weights

Cleaning and maintenance

Cleaning supplies needed:

_____ Four spray bottles (use one solely for water, the others for disinfectant and mark the bottles accordingly)

_____ Paper towels

_____ Cloth towels and hand rags

_____ Antibacterial cleaning spray

_____ Window and mirror cleaner

_____ Small vacuum cleaner

_____ Mop and bucket

Maintenance supplies needed:

_____ Pliers (standard and needlenose)

_____ Screwdrivers (standard and Phillips)

_____ Allen wrench set

_____ Crescent wrench

_____ Lubricant spray

_____ Socket set

Cardiovascular equipment cleaning schedule:

Daily

_____ Clean electronic consoles with plain water and a clean cloth

_____ Clean exterior of machines with disinfectant and a clean cloth

Monthly

_____ Treadmills: Remove the cover and vacuum the motor electronic compartment

_____ Treadmills: Check the belt tension and tracking. Check the amperage draw to ensure that it is within the manufactures requirements. Raise the elevation and vacuum underneath the treadmill

_____ Ellipicals: Remove the motor cover and vacuum the area surrounding the generator

_____ Bikes: Remove the cover and vacuum the motor electronic compartment

Quarterly

_____ Stepmill: Cleaning and lubrication internal components are required. Calling a specialist is recommended

Resistance training equipment cleaning schedule:

Daily:

_____ Wipe down upholstery with disinfectant and inspect it for tears

Weekly:

_____ Clean frames with disinfectant

_____ Check cables for proper tension

_____ Make sure weight collars fit snugly and examine the weight plates for any cracks

_____ Clean mirrors and glass surfaces

Monthly:

_____ Inspect cables and handgrips for wear

_____ Lubricate guide rods with Teflon spray. Never use WD-40 as a lubricant because it is a part cleaner and will remove all the lubrication from the rods

_____ Check the bolts, screws and adjustment mechanisms on dumbbells, racks and benches

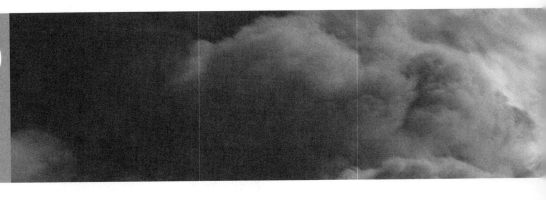

Appendix D
FIREFIGHTER FITNESS RESOURCES

Books:

- Collins, Jim, PhD. *Good to Great*. Harper Collins. New York, NY. 2001.

- Davids, Keith, Button, Chris, & Bennett, Simon. *Dynamics of Skill Acquisition*. Human Kinetics Publications, Champaign, IL. 2008.

- Orlick, Terry, PhD. *In Pursuit of Excellence*. 4th ed. Human Kinetics Publications, Champaign, IL, 2008.

- Murphy, Shane, *The Sport Psych Handbook*. Human Kinetics Publications, Champaign, IL. 2005.

- Jackson, Susanna, & Csikszentmihalyi, Mihaly. *Flow in Sports-The keys to optimal experiences and performances*, Human Kinetics Publications, Champaign, IL. 1999.

- Nelson, Arnold, PhD, & Kokkonen, Jouko, PhD. *Stretching Anatomy*. Human Kinetics Publications, Champaign, IL. 2000.

- Roizen, Michael, MD. *The Real Age Diet*, Harper Collins Publishers, New York, NY. 2001.

- Kleiner, Susan, PhD, RD. & Greenwood-Robinson, Maggie, PhD. *Power Eating*. 2nd Ed. Human Kinetics Publications, Champaign, IL. 2001.

- Boyle, Mike, MS. *Functional Training for Sports*. Human Kinetics Publications, Champaign, IL. 2004.

- Delavier, Fredric. *Strength Training Anatomy*. Human Kinetics Publications, Champaign, IL. 2001.

- Bompa, Tudor, PhD, & Carrera, Mike, MS. *Periodization Training for Sports*, 2nd Edition. Human Kinetics Publications, Champaign, IL. 2005.

- Fleck, Steve, PhD & Kraemer, William, PhD. *Periodization Breakthrough!* Advanced Research Press, Ronkonkoma, NY. 1996.

- ACSM's Guidelines for Exercise Testing and Prescription, 7th edition, Lippincott, Williams & Wilkins, Philadelphia, PA. May, 2005.

- Heyward, Vivian, PhD. *Advanced Fitness Assessment and Exercise Prescription*. 5th Edition. Human Kinetics, Champaign, IL. 2006.

- *Essentials of Strength Training and Conditioning, National Strength & Conditioning Association*. 3rd Edition, Human Kinetics, Champaign, IL. 2008.

- McGill, Stuart, PhD. *Low Back Disorders*. 2nd Edition, Human Kinetics, Champaign, IL. 2007.

- Fleck, Steve, PhD, & Kraemer, William, PhD. *Optimizing Strength Training. Designing Nonlinear Periodization Workouts*. Human Kinetics, Champaign, IL. 2007.

Websites:

American Council on Exercise (ACE), www.acefitness.org

American College of Sports Medicine (ACSM), www.acsm.org

National Strength & Conditioning Association (NSCA), www.nsca-lift.org

United States Fire Administration, Health and Safety, https://www.usfa.dhs.gov/fireservice/subjects/health/index.shtm

National Institute for Occupational Safety and Health, www.cdc.gov/niosh/fire

International Association of Fire Chiefs Health and Safety Section, www.iafcsafety.org

International Association of Fire Fighters Health and Safety, www.iaff.org/hs/index.htm

National Fallen Firefighters Foundation, www.firehero.org

National Fire Protection Association, www.nfpa.org

National Volunteer Fire Council Heart Healthy Firefighter, www.healthy-firefighter.org

National Interagency Fire Center, Fire Fit Program, www.nifc.gov/FireFit/index.htm

United States Department of Agriculture, My Pyramid, www.mypyramid.gov

Periodicals:

The Journal of Strength and Conditioning Research, Lippincott, Williams & Wilkins, Philadelphia, PA

Strength & Conditioning Journal, National Strength & Conditioning Association. Lippincott, Williams & Wilkins, Philadelphia, PA

ACSM's *Health & Fitness Journal*, Lippincott, Williams & Wilkins, Philadelphia, PA

IDEA Fitness Journal, IDEA Fitness & Health Inc. San Diego, CA

Training & Conditioning, MAG intl. Ithaca, NY

Equipment Dealers:

Perform Better-MF Athletic, PO Box 8090, Cranston, RI 02920-0090

800-556-7464 www.performbetter.com

Power Systems, PO Box 51030, Knoxville, TN 37950-1030

800-321-6975 www.power-systems.com

Country Technology, Inc. PO Box 87, Gays Mills, WI 54631

608-735-4718 www.fitnessmart.com

Index